7 Things You Must Know Before You Have Plastic Surgery:

1. Your Doctor, his training, skills and style

2. The surgical facility and who's really doing the surgery

3. The games and scams that doctors and their offices play

4. What can cause us to make good or bad decisions and how to trust your intuition.

5. The procedures, their benefits, and what really can go wrong

6. How to recognize that something is wrong

7. When to get a second opinion and how to get help

Published by Motivational Press, Inc.
2360 Corporate Circle
Suite 400
Henderson, NV 89074
www.MotivationalPress.com

www.TrustMeImAPlasticSurgeon.com

Manufactured in the United States of America.

ISBN: 978-1628650013

Trust Me, I'm a Plastic Surgeon
The Survival Guide

By
Donald W. Kress, M.D., F.A.C.S.

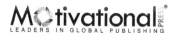
M⊙tivational PRESS ®
LEADERS IN GLOBAL PUBLISHING

Contents

Dedication

First, I would like to dedicate this book to my sister Cheryl. She was the brightest and most capable of three children, but growing up without a mother was especially difficult for her. She died much too young and before she was able to pass on to the world her compassion, insights and humanity. From those of us who really knew her, we will never stop missing her.

Second, I would like to dedicate this book to all of the injured and disappointed people who paid good money to feel better about themselves by having Plastic Surgery, only to have it go embarrassingly wrong. My hope is that this book will give you the knowledge and courage to get the help you need. For those contemplating Plastic Surgery, I hope the information in this book helps you to better understand the processes, the procedures and the players, in order for you to make better decisions and avoid the pain and embarrassment of bad Plastic Surgery.

Finally, I would like to dedicate this to my mentor, William P Graham III for teaching me the skills of Plastic Surgery, and, perhaps more importantly, for passing on his integrity, compassion, work ethic, and his endless passion for improving the specialty.

Acknowledgements

To Ann McIndoo, my author's coach who not only helped me get this book out of my head and onto paper, but cheered me on with her perpetual good humor, encouragement, and optimism.

To my wife Kimberly who realized early, the importance of this book, helped with the editing, offered encouragement, and never complained about all the time I took away from us to spend on the book.

To my artist daughter, Kimberly, for all her help designing the cover, illustrating the book, and lending encouragement.

To my office staff, Ceejae Bennett, Allison Grant, Charity Riggs, and Sharon Sanbower, who adjusted my schedule, helped me organize the patient photos, looked up journal articles for me and did some amazing adjustments to the office schedule to accommodate the project.

Author's Note

When I first began my career in Plastic Surgery over 30 years ago. I rarely saw bad results from Plastic Surgery problems. That doesn't mean they didn't occur but I suspect that the conscientious surgeons fixed their own problems. "Even good surgeons have things go wrong", what defines them as good surgeons is the determination to stay with the patient until the best possible outcome is achieved.

Over the years, three things changed. The number of untrained or poorly trained doctors doing plastic surgery has steadily increased. The number of problems or complications has increased. And, most importantly, the number of injured patients desperate to find help for their problems has increased.

As I experienced the numbers of these injured patients gradually rise from two per year to over 20% of my practice, I was struck by the fact the patients really didn't know how to prepare for and qualify their doctor, and intuitively they knew that something would go wrong.

Taking care of injured patients has its own special difficulties. They have already spent a lot of money, they are uncertain how to get out of the injury cycle without risking additional injury, they are leery of trying to qualify another doctor when the first choice didn't work out, and they're angry. It's no wonder than many Plastic Surgeons don't want to deal with them. Like my patient with an infected tummy tuck done in Ecuador, she had seen 5 plastic surgeons who all refused to care for her before coming to me.

I decided at this stage of my career to take care of the injured patients as best I could by offering good surgical care and sympathy. I also realized that in order to reverse this trend I would have to write a book. "Trust Me I'm a Plastic Surgeon" will teach anyone how to prepare for surgery, recognize their own weaknesses and vulnerabilities, evaluate the doctors, facilities, procedures, and the decision process. I also offer advice on how and when to get help if something does go wrong. The book may offend some of the medical societies and doctors but it's based on consultations with literally hundreds of injured patients and my reflection of what could have helped them to make better decisions.

Better decisions equal better outcomes!

Foreword

My previous Doctor *disfigured my breasts. I had seven surgeries by the same Doctor, each time he promised to make them better but instead I got worse each time. I heard of Dr. Kress and went to see if he could correct them. I am VERY happy with the results. Dr. Kress and his staff are phenomenal!!! Exquisite attention to detail!!!*

PH

After going to another Doctor for a breast lift and an implant, I was very dissatisfied with the results and several attempts at correction. I chose to come to Dr. Kress in the hopes he could make me look as normal as possible. He did a corrective lift and used gel implants to replace the saline ones I had already. He was pleasant and very honest as to what he could do to repair what had been done by the previous Doctor. I am so happy I found him and he made me feel like a brand new woman. I wish I had found him sooner. Thank you Dr. Kress.

SF

I would like to, once again, thank you for giving me back my appearance of 10 years ago, or even more.

I would also like to share a couple of thoughts with you. It is my belief that for a good surgeon it is mandatory to have skillful hands that can master the scalpel, excellent knowledge of anatomy, and a sharp mind that can make life-depending decisions in seconds. A good plastic surgeon however, especially one who performs face work, must possess attributes way beyond that. A plastic surgeon must also have the eye and the soul of an artist. He needs to have the feel, the touch and the talent of a sculptor. What else is a face-lift if not sculpturing? And, in my view, it is the most masterful of all sculpturing arts, since the carving has to be done into the most demanding of all sculpturing materials – the human flesh.

What a shame it is that, while Michelangelo's sculptures in marble will forever remain to delight the senses of mortals, your masterpieces are as ephemeral as the human life itself...Well, my husband and my daughter will definitely enjoy one of your masterpieces for a while!

And would you like me to tell you when was the time I discovered the fact that you were not only an excellent surgeon but also and extremely talented artist? It was

9

the moment I noticed that, while all other plastic surgeons would draw some guiding lines on your face prior to surgery, you have not done that. That very moment I Knew you were not just the regular surgeon who would simply follow standard operating procedures without necessarily having in mind what the exact outcome would be, but you were rather the artist who would use his talent and creativity to step by step reconstruct my youthful look. And, that was exactly what you have done, and the outcome was exactly the one I hoped for. My face looks exactly as it did ten, even more than ten years ago. And for that, I do not know how I should thank you other than simply saying: THANK YOU! Sincerely,

DC

Part I
Introduction

Beauty: The adjustment of all parts proportionately so that one cannot add or subtract or change without impairing the harmony of the whole.
--Leon Battista Alberti

What is Plastic Surgery and where did it come from?

What is beauty?

Can it be defined?

Is beauty universal, cultural, individual or all of these?

What is the effect of the media on the "standard of beauty"?

Is that bad?

Why would anyone write this book anyway?

Plastic surgery was born during the course of WWI in England, to deal with the soldiers suffering mutilating facial injuries. The father of plastic surgery, Sir Harold Gilles, was an Otolaryngologist (Ear, Nose and Throat Doctor) who joined the Royal Army Medical Corps at the start of the War. After working with several famous Dentists and Maxillofacial surgeons, he learned their techniques of skin grafting and jaw reconstruction. He returned to England in 1917 and persuaded the Army's chief surgeon to establish a facial injury ward, which expanded so quickly it had to be moved to the Queen's Hospital. There, over the years, Sir Harold and his colleagues developed many of the techniques now known as Plastic Surgery. They performed over 11,000 operations on 5,000 men (mostly soldiers with facial injuries). Sir Harold Gilles was knighted in 1930. Between WW I and WW II, Sir Harold continued to develop new procedures. Many of the founders of the specialty trained with Sir Harold and later took these techniques and principles around the world.

The word "plastic" doesn't mean plastic in the sense that we now know it (toy trucks and kitchen tools); the word plastic is derived from a Greek word plastikos, which means, "to mold". Unfortunately, when the term Plastic Surgery came into use, no one thought to patent or restrict the term itself and now, unfortunately, the number and variety of surgeons using the term "Plastic Surgeon" to describe themselves and the number of organizations including the term "Plastic Surgery" is in the dozens.

The origins of modern Plastic Surgery started with the deformities of war injuries, but prior to this a 16th century barber surgeon named Gaspar Tagliacozzi had already developed many techniques for nasal reconstruction. Some of which are still used. Rebuilding amputated noses from dueling or punishment was a challenging and rewarding use of skills that would later be incorporated into Plastic Surgery. In his early publications he said; "We restore, rebuild and make whole that parts . . . which nature has given but which fortune has taken away, not so much that it might delight the eye but it might buoy up the spirit and help the mind of the beset."

It did not take long for creative doctors to apply these reconstructive techniques and principles to other patients who wanted correction for deformities of birth or the effects of aging and the field of "Cosmetic Surgery" was born. Likewise, it didn't take long for the charlatans, frauds, pretenders and fakes to emerge with unproven techniques, lack of training, illegal materials and dangerous substances to take advantage of those who failed to do their homework.

For perspective, in the year 2011 there were 13.8 million cosmetic procedures in the USA alone with a value of 10.4 billion dollars and 5.5 million reconstructive procedures. See www.plasticsurgery.org. The top cosmetic procedures in order are; Breast Augmentation, Nasal surgery, Liposuction, Eyelid surgery, and Facelift.

That pleasure which is at once the most pure, the most elevating,
and the most intense, is derived, I maintain, from the
contemplation of the beautiful.
--Edgar Allen Poe

Definitions of Beauty and the Changing Nature of Beauty

"To a toad, what is beauty?
A female with two pop-eyes, a wide mouth,
yellow belly and spotted back"
--Voltaire

"Attractive children are more popular, both with classmates and teachers; teachers give higher evaluations of the work of attractive children and have higher expectations of them, which have shown to improve performance. Attractive applicants have a better chance of getting jobs and receiving higher salaries. One US study found that taller men earned around $600 per inch more than shorter executives. In court, attractive people are found guilty less often; when found guilty they receive lighter sentences. The bias for beauty operates in all social circumstances; all experiments show we react more favorably to physically attractive people. We also believe in the, "what is beautiful is good" stereotype and an irrational deep-seated belief that physically attractive people possess other desirable characteristics such as intelligence, confidence, social skills and even moral virtue. "The good fairy princess is always beautiful, the wicked stepmother is always ugly."

http://www.sirc.org/publik/mirror.html Last accessed 9/5/2012

There is no question that cultural variations exist in the concept of beauty. There is an island in the Pacific where beautiful means that you have no front teeth. On that island, Tetanus or lockjaw, was a significant killer of children many generations ago. There was no treatment for tetanus or lockjaw. With all of their teeth and no way to give nutrition, if they developed lockjaw they would die of starvation. As a rite of passage, parents would pull their children's four front teeth. This allowed the children to be fed through the gap and survive in the event of Tetanus. Over time, people that were missing their front teeth became the standard of beauty for the island and now the islanders believe that people who have their full set of front teeth look dangerous and vicious.

In some Asian cultures it's common for people to believe that fat equals fertile and affluent. Fat women are especially desirable because the implication is that you have come from wealth and that you would be better able to produce children.

The Golden Ratio has, for over 1,200 years, been considered a standard of aesthetics for both faces and architecture. The ratio is a mathematical comparison of two adjacent areas and the ideal is 1 to 1.618. It has been referred to as "Phi" and this ratio was instrumental in paintings by Michelangelo, DaVinci and many others. The use of Phi is instrumental in architecture and the design of many famous buildings including the Parthenon and the pyramids.

Phi is a way of statistically measuring beauty by comparing size and ratios of eyes, lips, nose and the spaces between them. Dr. Stephen Marquardt, an oral and maxillofacial surgeon, has done extensive studies of Phi and it's application to beauty. He's developed a mathematical mask that can be overlaid on photos to evaluate beauty. When he applies the mask to the world's most beautiful people, they fit with uncanny accuracy. For less-than-perfect people, applying the mask to their photos can show where changes (sometimes quite small) can dramatically affect the perception of beauty. www.goldennumber.net/beauty

Critics of statistical methods for evaluation of beauty frequently refer to the famous old adage, "Beauty is in the Eye of the Beholder." Modern research and Dr. Marquardt challenge this notion. He finds that an ideal of beauty exists, and is not only cross-cultural but can be applied even to ancient concepts of beauty.

"Young infants are aware of attractiveness and exhibit preferences for attractive faces that mirror those of adults. Infants as young as a few days of age seem to prefer and look longer at faces adults judge to be attractive.

Averageness is the only characteristic discovered to date that is both necessary and sufficient to insure facial attractiveness. "Without a facial configuration close to the average of the population, a face will not be attractive no matter how smooth, youthful or symmetrical; averageness is fundamental." Does this averaging make the faces a better fit for Dr. Marquard's Phi-based mask?

> Rhodes, G., Zebrowitz, L.A.,(2002) *Facial Attractiveness; Evolutionary, Cognitive, and Social Perspectives.* Westport Connecticut, Ablex

In every computer model developed to study facial attractiveness, when researchers blend more than 16 faces together, the people doing the evaluations rate it as highly attractive. If more than 16 faces are blended together; the level of attractiveness increases still more. Contrary to the old adage about the "eye of the beholder", the results indicate a high level of agreement about attractiveness from even different types of raters (old, young, male, female and cross-cultural).

Media

Media manipulation of the concepts of beauty for their own gain invades nearly every aspect of our lives. To improve sales of products, fashion, cosmetics, and other gadgets, marketers from these industries have barraged us with images of the super model as the goal of the consumer. The typical model appearing in media represents a nearly unattainable image. Actually, less than two percent of women in the United States would be able to achieve the physical characteristics of a model.

A quote from the Body Project (helping young girls feel better about themselves with less than perfect bodies) states, "The average American woman is 5'4" and 140 pounds; the average fashion model is 5'11" and 115 pounds. Fashion models are thinner than 98% of American women. Eighty percent of women in the United States are dissatisfied with their appearance. Ninety percent of women in a recent survey on a college campus said they've attempted to control their weight through dieting. Twenty five percent of men and 45% of women are on a diet at any given time. Approximately seven million girls and women, and one million boys and men, struggle with eating disorders."

If Barbie was a real woman she would lack enough body fat to menstruate, her measurements would be 39-21-33, she would be six feet tall and weigh 100 pounds. In the average population, there is less than one chance in 100,000 of obtaining those numbers. The question then becomes, is it possible that the media is creating eating disorders and other problems with self-esteem by setting unattainable standards?

An experimental evaluation was conducted in the last decade on the island of Fiji. Prior to the introduction of American media, eating disorders were entirely unknown on Fiji. Within three years of the introduction of American media on local TV stations and in print, eating disorders began to emerge in Fiji.

There is no accountability of the media and the influences they have on the public, both American and international, but there have been some counter movements. *Vogue* magazine recently banned models that are either too thin or less than the age of 16.

Seventeen magazine's "*Seventeen* Body Peace Project" is a set of pledges for young women to better accept their natural beauty and to develop an appreciation for their differences. The *Dove* "Real Beauty Campaign" promotes true beauty of people of differing ages and figures. International modeling shows no longer employ models who don't meet the minimum BMI[G] (Body Mass Index) threshold.

It remains to be seen if these counter-culture movements will expand and gain wider acceptance, or if they themselves are just another media manipulation.

Why this book?

My reasons for writing this book are simple. Over thirty years of practice, I've watched the number of bad Plastic Surgery cases steadily increase. It's now so bad that I'm reluctant to visit some of our major cities. The number and extent of bad Plastic Surgery walking around the streets is painful to observe. I can't even go through the grocery store checkout without having to look at images of human caricatures on the magazine covers. One of our major meetings was opened by a distinguished professor of Plastic Surgery who said in his introductory remarks; "I've come to the conclusion that patient satisfaction must be 90% the charm of the doctor, or how else can you explain all of the bad Plastic Surgery walking around?" Some of the bad Plastic Surgery comes from unqualified doctors, some come from unscrupulous doctors, some come from untrained doctors, some come from having the wrong procedure, but all of them come from making bad decisions.

Ultimately, if you decide to have Plastic Surgery, you will make the decision of what, with whom, where and how to have Plastic Surgery. It's my job and the purpose of this book to give you the tools you need to make those decisions better.

"How can you get very far,
If you don't know who you are?
How can you do what you ought,
If you don't know what you've got?
And if you don't know which to do
Of all the things in front of you,
Then what you'll have when you are through
Is just a mess without a clue
Of all the best that can come true
If you know What and Which and Who."
*--**Benjamin Hoff, The Tao of Pooh***

Trust Me, I'm a Plastic Surgeon

Chapter One
The Doctor

The auto mechanic says to the heart surgeon,
"I fix your car's engine and get paid three hundred dollars.
You fix a human engine and get paid twenty times that.
Why is that?"
Heart surgeon, "Try fixing the car's engine while it's running."

What's a medical student, an intern, a resident and a chief resident?

How do they get where they are?

What are "Board Eligible" and "Board Certified"

Who exactly is a Plastic Surgeon and what are their societies?

What are the alternative boards?

How do Plastic Surgeons keep up their skills and education?

Are the dates of the Plastic Surgery meetings important?

What kinds of Plastic Surgeons are there?

What effect does the Media have on Plastic Surgery.

What if you're rejected by a Plastic Surgeon?

Who's watching the doctors?

To know more about Plastic Surgery and Plastic Surgeons, it's helpful to understand their training, their certification and how they keep current (or not). First, because it helps to understand the way they think, and second, if you are ever a patient in a teaching institution, it can be really helpful to know whom you're talking to.

Medical School, Students, and "Match Day"

The lowest person in the medical pecking order is the medical student in his third or fourth year of medical school. This person is not yet a doctor in the sense they haven't passed any boards or been licensed by any state. Traditional medical education is frequently divided into two classroom years and two clinical years. In some teaching facilities, you can identify the medical student by the length or color of coat they wear (you may have to ask them). Medical student in the clinical years rotate among the principle medical specialties (Ob-Gyn, Surgery, Internal Medicine, ER, Radiology, Pathology and more). They learn clinical techniques, observe and assist in medical procedures and participate in decision-making. Hopefully, during these rotations, he/she will find an area that has a special appeal. Don't be surprised if a medical student takes an hour to do your history and physical only to have it repeated by someone higher in the pecking order. (Be Patient! Everyone has to start somewhere.) Certain personality types will predictably gravitate to the specialties that fit them. The surgeons tend to be aggressive, and immediate gratification people versus the internists who are problem solvers. Internists can take weeks, multiple tests, and treatment trials to solve their medical puzzles.

After graduation, they can add M.D. to their name. Prior to graduation they visit potential residency programs in their chosen specialties. The program directors interview the candidates and the students take a look at the facilities and the program to see if there's a match. The students turn in a list of their choices and the program directors turn in their choices to the matching agency. On a magic day actually called "Match Day", letters go out to the students with offers of residencies. Some programs are highly competitive with dozens more applicants than they can accept. If you've applied to several programs (a good idea!) "Match Day" can be exciting. Not quite the NFL draft but similar. On that day the soon-to-be doctor will learn the direction of their career and where they're going to spend the next two to seven years.

Medical License

Near the conclusion of Medical School, the future doctors undergo standard testing. The scores are sent to the states they're considering. Licenses are state issued; with a lot of variability in the requirements and maintenance of the license. Florida, for example, has a reputation for having a challenging licensing exam (they write their own). Once a Florida license is granted, however, Florida is lax in monitoring what type of specialist the Doctors choose to call themself. State societies have the primary responsibility of monitoring the activities of their Doctors, keeping licenses current, evaluating complaints of substance abuse, illegal activities, malpractice claims and complaints in general. All states have disciplinary boards, which can be a good source of information when you're checking on a Doctor.

Residency/Intern

The concept of "intern" is still used but dates back to the days when general practitioners (GP's) would do an internship and then go into community practice. Now, it just refers to the first year of residency.

To go into the specialty of Plastic Surgery, you must first complete a residency in General Surgery, which is usually five years. In the "olden days" Surgical residencies were a lot like fraternity hazing. Days without sleep, constantly being questioned about decisions, and a lot of hard work. It was not unusual to leave home at five am and not return for three days. Was this necessary to train a future surgeon, or was it a test of endurance? Now that most programs have been "humanized", it remains to be seen if we produce the same caliber of surgeons.

Having undergone the rigorous surgical residency, I think it is probably an excellent preparation for life as a surgeon. It exposes the future surgeon to the drama of middle-of-the-night trauma and life or death situations. One definition of a surgeon is "a doctor who is able to make life-and-death decisions with completely inadequate information".

A senior Plastic Surgeon that I worked with for years tells the story of arriving at John's Hopkins for his first day of residency. He was nicely dressed and was given his first pager and his ID badge. The pager went off and told him to go immediately to the emergency room. When he finally found the emergency room and the person who paged him, it was another resident who had a patient's chest open and his hand inside massaging the heart to keep the patient alive. The resident told him; "They're coming to take him to the operating room in a few minutes. I'm late for my next rotation. Put on gloves and take over for me." You can easily imagine what he looked like after this adventure.

This kind of training teaches the surgeon to remain calm, analyze the situation and take charge no matter how bad the emergency. Have you ever seen a surgeon jump up and down because he won a contest or had a perfect hole of golf? I used to go deep-sea fishing yearly, and the captain would sometimes comment, "you just caught a great fish, why aren't you excited?" The answer is that, "I am excited on the inside, but in my business it isn't good to show too much excitement or the people around me might think I'm not in control." Although these experiences are rare in the world of Plastic Surgery, the lessons learned, like riding a bike, are never forgotten and will re-emerge even years later in the event of a serious emergency. (This is the first of many reasons why you should consider carefully one of the "alternatively credentialed Plastic Surgeons" who bypassed or was unable to qualify for this part of their training.)

The board certifying agencies require that all residencies include progressive responsibility (both the surgical cases and the decision making) under the direction of the residency program director. Plastic Surgeons do this twice. They first complete a general surgery program (5 years) with the final year as a Chief Resident and then go through the system again (and the match) for their Plastic Surgery Residency with another year as a Chief Resident (2 years minimum). There are occasions that completion of another surgical residency such as otolaryngology or neurosurgery will be admitted to a Plastic Surgery Training Program.

Chief Resident

The Chief Resident is in his/her final year of training and has achieved sufficient status and experience to be treated as a staff member (almost). The staff are all board certified Plastic Surgeons, many with super-specialties, working in the Department, doing research, running clinics within the institution, seeing patients, operating and supervising the training programs. By this stage, most Chief Residents have adopted a "mentor" or one of the senior staff with which they have a special bond. This mentor does a lot to shape the "style" of the new Plastic Surgeon. My mentor, William P Graham, was an internationally famous Plastic Surgery educator. Thirty years later I can still hear him whispering in my ear from time to time. "OK, you've got plan A, but what about plan B and C." "All surgery has one or two things to accomplish and one or two things to avoid (the dragons), remember what they are and get on with it!" "There is no such thing as *simple* surgery! There are only, *simple* surgeons."

If you decide to have your surgery done at a teaching hospital, you're going to meet the people who will actually do the surgery. The "attending" is the staff surgeon who will be responsible for your surgery, make the decisions, and decide who will assist and to what degree they assist. If the surgery is difficult or if the residents don't have enough experience, the attending will do the actual surgery. A beginning resident will be doing some wound closures, surgical cleaning of wounds or burns (debridement), emergency room repair of lacerations, etc. Remember that a beginning resident in Plastic Surgery is already a fully qualified General Surgeon. The Chief Resident will be developing treatment plans and executing surgical procedures in consultation with his "attending" staff.

Board Eligible

Before finishing the residency program the Chief Resident in Plastic Surgery must satisfactorily pass the first of two board exams. The Program Director will then sign a letter to the board attesting to the satisfactory completion of his/her training. The new Plastic Surgeon will now enter practice by; joining a group, setting up a solo practice, joining an academic team, or completing a military obligation. He/she is now able to call themselves "Board Eligible". When you're checking on a potential doctor, you now know what that term means.

It will be nearly a year in practice with extensive documentation of all of their procedures, results, and safety practices before they can move on to an even more difficult oral exam and case review. Satisfactory completion of that exam allows a surgeon to use the term "Board Certified". Board Certification in the United States is voluntary but most of the major hospitals will give the new doctor a few years grace to complete their board requirements or else they can withdraw privileges.

Board Certified

We have arrived at an important category. What exactly is "Board Certification"? The American Board of Medical Specialties[A] (ABMS) is the oldest and most respected medical specialty-certifying agency. Through their 24 member boards, they:

- Evaluate and monitor the training programs for residents. They have the power to withdraw certification if they feel the program is not meeting the standards.

- Establish requirements for the qualification of applicants.

- Conduct examinations of approved candidates who seek certification.

- Issue certificates to those who meet the requirements and pass the exams.

- Establish minimal requirements of continuing education to maintain the certification.

Of the 24 member boards of the ABMS only one of these, called the "American Board of Plastic Surgery[A] "(ABPS), is involved with the training and certification of Plastic Surgeons. Competency is defined by the ABPS[A] as "an amalgam of basic medical and surgical knowledge, operative judgment, technical expertise, ethical behavior and interpersonal skills to achieve problem resolution and patient satisfaction. All of this insures a uniform and high level of resident training and reassurance to the public of the quality of education and training."

There are two problems with this system. First, most states do not require a practitioner to specify which of the 24 boards he/she is certified in. It isn't unusual for a gynecologist, who is finding his income dropping, to start doing liposuction for a little bit of extra cash. He/she is able to advertise as "Board Certified", but not required to say which board. Is it an appropriate board? Certainly in Florida, if your surgeon is a board certified Podiatrist (foot doctor), you should think twice about having this doctor do your breast implants.

Alternative Boards (not recognized by the ABMS[A])

The second problem is the doctors claiming "board certification" (alternative boards) in a board not recognized by ABMS. Many of these "alternative boards" have official and impressive sounding names. Some even claim they are more specialized and have superior surgeons than the Plastic Surgeons because they have the word "face" or "cosmetic" in their name. They're not monitored, evaluated or examined by the ABMS and make their own rules. Their requirements for admission and ongoing membership vary considerably from the American Board of Plastic Surgery. Some of these "alternative boards" validate themselves by declaring that they sit on a council of the AMA. The AMA is a voluntary organization for all physicians and it does not qualify anybody to be a cosmetic or Plastic Surgeon. The American Board of Otolaryngology, which is certified by the ABMS, monitors the education and certifies some excellent cosmetic surgeons. Their training is limited to the face, head, and neck. In those areas they can become masters. When they expand their practices to other body areas, breast, liposuction, and tummy tucks, there may be problems.

There may be excellent surgeons who, for various reasons, have chosen to take a non-certified route, perhaps because they were unwilling to take the time, they couldn't qualify, or they were not even in a surgical specialty. Outside of the ABPS these surgeons have widely varying levels of training and experience. When evaluating a doctor, ask two questions; "Are you Board Certified?" and What Board are you certified by?" Yes, and the American Board of Plastic Surgery are your safest answers.

I was clearing mail from my desk after being out of town for a few days and ran across an ad from one of the impressive sounding "alternative associations". This organization was offering a three-hour course in Florida featuring a "World Famous Surgeon" who would teach the attendees all they needed to know about breast augmentation; presumably, so that they could return home and incorporate this into their practice. To put that into perspective, by the time I completed my training and started to do breast augmentations, I had done, participated in, or watched over 300 breast augmentations including many "problem" cases.

IMPORTANT NOTE

You probably aren't interested in being overwhelmed by the alphabet soup of all these organizations. Your interest is in making certain that you have the safest and best possible surgery. Board certification is important but only one part of the picture. It certainly will help you weed-out some of the pretenders and complete frauds.

If you read the publications from our societies, they imply that Board Certification is sufficient to ensure an excellent and safe procedure. I've seen injuries, scams, and dreadful results from Board Certified Plastic Surgeons. And, I've seen beautifully elegant facial work by ENT Plastic Surgeons. I have a lot more you need to know, and as Mr. Filch said in Harry Potter; "You're going to have to keep your wits about you."

More Alphabet Soup

Sorry, but there are some other organizations you'll encounter that are important and only allow membership to Board Certified Plastic Surgeons.

ABPS (The American Board of Plastic Surgery[A]) – This is the organization responsible for the Plastic surgery training programs.

ASPS (The American Society of Plastic Surgeons[A]) – The parent organization of practicing Board certified Plastic Surgeons. Virtually all Plastic Surgeons belong to this organization. The society has a membership, voting body, code of ethics, an ethics review panel, and dozens of committees. They also establish continuing education requirements, recertification examinations (with ABPS) and organize several annual educational meetings.

ASAPS (The American Society for Aesthetic Plastic Surgery[A]) – A specialist society for Plastic Surgeons who's practice is primarily aesthetic or cosmetic. They organize educational opportunities focused on the interests and needs of their members, the Aesthetic Surgeons.

ISAPS (The International Society of Aesthetic Plastic Surgery[A]) – Similar to ASAPS but encouraging leaders from around the world to become members and share global concepts of Aesthetics and Aesthetic Surgery.

Within the broad field of Plastic Surgery there are societies that focus on hands, micro-surgery, facial deformities, use of fat grafting, burns, lasers, and more.

IMPORTANT NOTE

The American Society of Plastic Surgeons has a strict Code of Ethics about fees, practices, and advertising. The content of any ad (including the internet) must be fully verifiable. Member Plastic Surgeons cannot make statements of the "best", "most up to date", "most experienced", "most effective", or any claim that cannot be proven and fully documented

The "alternative" specialty boards and Societies have much less stringent Ethics. The explosive growth of the Internet and social media has made the problem even worse. If you're browsing the Internet or even traveling down the highway and run across the "Best Plastic Surgery in --------", you can be certain that this is not a member of ASPS.

Meetings and Continuing Education

There are a few things to know about the meetings, conferences and continuing education programs for plastic surgeons. The ASPS has stringent requirements for keeping up member's education. They require almost four weeks of educational activities every two years including patient safety issues.

The biggest conference of the year, the American Society of Plastic Surgeons, usually occurs in the fall. Upwards of 5,000 US Plastic Surgeons attend this meeting. This is the general Plastic Surgery society and topics range from the latest in burn care, cranio-facial malformations, skin cancer, and of course, cosmetic surgery. There are focused sessions where Doctors or researchers on a specific techniques or topics present their findings. There are sessions of general interest to all Plastic Surgeons as well as teaching courses. Last, but not least, there is a trade-show area where manufacturers of Plastic Surgery gizmos and gadgets show off their latest and greatest.

In addition to the Society meetings, there are annual specialty meetings on specific topics. In Atlanta and Santa Fe there are annual meetings entirely devoted to body contouring and breast surgery. A surgeon can easily attend a meeting with three full days of the latest and most up to date information on breast surgery, surgery after weight reduction, liposuction, noses or others.

The second largest meeting of the year is the ASAPS[G] meeting usually held in May. This meeting is focused entirely on the cosmetic or aesthetic side of Plastic Surgery.

The Danger of Meetings and Why Those Dates Are Important

One of the real dangers, and why it is important to know the dates, is the documented increase in the number and type of surgical complications following one of these meetings. The explanation is thought to relate to younger surgeons who return home from the meeting and attempt the techniques they saw presented at the meeting often with less than satisfactory results. More experienced surgeons are comfortable working a little further from the "front edge" of the specialty and prefer to introduce new ideas into their practice a little at a time or to wait to see if this is new technique is a dead end or the beginning of a real breakthrough. One of my first partners was convinced that liposuction (now Plastic Surgery's number two procedure) was never going to last and that all the fat would just come back. It took me years of convincing to get him to pick up a cannula and see for himself.

Since we're discussing dates to watch out for, mention must be made of the first of July. EVERYTHING in medicine changes on the first of July. New Doctors go into practice, new residents start their residencies, older residents are promoted to the next level, and doctors in training rotate onto services they've never seen before. This can be a dangerous week to go to the emergency room.

Plastic Surgery Style

There are two main types of Plastic Surgeons. At the risk of gross over-simplification, I'll describe them as mechanical or artistic. Mechanical surgeons tend to be engineering types, who, once they learn a procedure and become proficient at getting a good and predictable result will not vary it. I have known surgeons who have been in practice for over 20 years that were still doing the exact same type and placement of sutures that their mentor taught them 20 years previously. Some famous Plastic Surgeons have been mechanical and achieved their fame from consistently excellent results

On the other hand, there are surgeons that I call artistic. Every time they do a case they try to think of ways to improve it. They are the innovators, who enjoy modifying a procedure to fit the particular nuances of a patient's needs, versus fitting the patient to a procedure with a consistently good outcome. Both have their place and both can have consistently good outcomes. When you're evaluating your potential doctor and listening to the proposed treatment plan, you may get a sense of the Doctor's style. You can also tell by looking at the photo albums. It has been said that a famous Philadelphia Plastic Surgeon made all of his noses look exactly the same, and they could be recognized from the opposite side of the road. Fine, if you like that model, not so good if you want your specific concerns addressed.

Another consideration is whether the surgeon is conservative verses "cutting edge". If you're the kind of person who sees something on Good Morning America and runs out to find someone to do it, you may be a little bit too close to the cutting edge.

I've known some extraordinarily good and conservative Plastic Surgeons that waited years before incorporate new technology into their practice. I've known others that were too close to the front edge and got involved in procedures that turned out to not be as effective as hoped. One innovative laser surgeon published some elegant papers on treating stretch marks with a new kind of laser. Two years after publishing the initial papers, she had to apologize to the Plastic Surgeon community. Most of the treated stretch marks had come back. Cellulite treatments, skin tightening, non-invasive liposuction, and thread-lifts to name just a few, have all had a brief moment of fame only to fade away.

When interviewing a doctor, if the proposed procedure is unfamiliar to you or suspicious, ask:

How long has this procedure been performed?

How many have you done?

How long is the follow-up on the patients?

Impact of Media

Media's insatiable appetite for all things newer, faster, better, and easier is hard on practicing Plastic Surgeons. Media has the ability to make an unproven technique or procedure (usually a new gadget) sound like the new "Gold Standard" of Plastic Surgery. You are being barraged daily with information from commercials, TV programs, infomercials, magazines and the web. Many people who call my office are convinced they just heard or saw the latest miracle in Plastic Surgery. It takes literally hours a week to answer these queries. My personal favorite is the housewife from New Jersey who discovered how to make herself 20 years younger. "Just call us and we'll let you in on 'the secret

Plastic Surgeons don't want you to know"'. And I thought falling for an email from Africa asking for your bank account numbers in order to send you your inherited millions from a long lost relative was dumb.

In the past, educated sales representatives went to doctors offices, brought samples, and explained the advantages of a new product. Now with new federal regulations, that type of physician education is nearly gone. Media doesn't miss a step. They took the product, the gadget or the drug directly to the consumer. Better to have the patients going into the doctor's office, "Hey Doc, I need those purple prostate pills so I can pee better." There are so many erectile dysfunction ads you might begin to wonder if anyone over the age of 50 could have sex without a pill. Plastic Surgery is not immune; marketers have taken some marginal devices and techniques directly to the consumer and promoted them in ways that our Code of Ethics would never allow. Now "no-cutting liposuction, cellulite cures, and scarless facelifts are mixed in with vacuums, pet brushes and beer commercials. If you're a new Plastic Surgeon and your office gets a dozen phone calls asking for a new fat removal device you might seriously consider getting one even though you heard at the last meeting that it doesn't work.

Remember what you're looking at. Although there is good medical educational programming, the goal of marketing is SALES not EDUCATION.

> *"Believe only half of what you see and nothing that you hear."*
> **—Edgar Allan Poe**

> *"Caveat Emptor." (Let the buyer beware.)*
> **--Latin Proverb**

Rejection

It's important to realize that a conscientious surgeon needs to reject some of the patients coming for consults. My old mentor used to say if you are not rejecting one out of every eight patients that come into your office, you are not doing your job, or your a service to the patients. I tell my patients that when someone who earns their living by doing surgery says you shouldn't have surgery, Listen!

There are a lot of reasons why you might find yourself referred for another evaluation or rejected:

- Unrealistic expectations – thinking that the procedure will do more than it can or there are too many risks for the potential gain.
- Poor physical condition.
- A health condition incompatible with significant surgery – Many Plastic Surgeons now include smoking in there along with blood thinners, poorly controlled diabetes, and heart conditions.
- Failure to establish a good doctor/patient relationship – sometimes the fit just isn't right.
- The procedure may not even be possible.

Danger – If you're rejected by a qualified Plastic Surgeon and continue to shop around, you'll eventually find someone who will do what you want. The results of this action are likely to be disappointing at best and fatal at the worst.

Who's Watching the Doctors

People believe that there are internal checks and balances that prevent bad doctors from practicing. That turns out to be true but not always effective. Each state has primary responsibility for their licensed physicians. Complaints about inappropriate physician behavior are investigated thoroughly and can lead to sanctions, or suspensions if the accusations are well founded. Unless somebody initiates the complaint, a bad or impaired doctor can practice for a long time below the radar. In one major eastern city, a surgeon's wife had to report her husband to the state board twice when his drug problem got so out-of-control she was afraid he would kill someone.

The specialty boards enforce their respective codes of ethics but they're primarily concerned with fees, advertising and marketing practices. The FDA, theoretically, is watching over doctors for controlled substance dispensing and the use of unapproved medical devices. But, again, without specific complaints abuses would be unlikely to come to their attention. In my community, one physician who told everyone he was doing well in the stock market was allegedly found to be selling narcotics prescriptions out of his office. Put the cash on the counter and pick up your prescription. This went on for years without detection.

As a patient, you have to look out for yourself, do your investigating, and if you encounter an impaired physician, report them to the state, their specialty society, or the FDA(see appendix). You may save someone's life or at least save them considerable pain and suffering.

A famous psychologist finding himself lecturing to a large auditorium full of practicing physicians, asked his audience to raise their hand if they personally knew a doctor who should not be practicing. EVERY hand went up.

Chapter Two
The Facilities

Life is short, the art long, opportunity fleeting, experiment treacherous, judgment difficult.
--Hippocrates

How do hospitals and clinics qualify their Doctors?

Can I save money going to a University Clinic?

What's a free standing Surgical Center?

How does the surgical schedule work?

Do I need to be concerned about who's doing anesthesia?

Can I save money going out of the country?

Hospitals

Now that you have some knowledge about Doctors, their Societies and their training, you also need to know about the facilities used for surgery, what happens there and the things that can go wrong.

What are *"admitting privilege"* or *"privilege's"* and what do these terms mean? For a physician to receive admitting privileges or to receive privileges in general, a physician has to go to a hospital, ask to become a member of the staff (pay a fee, of course) and indicate which procedures they would like to do at that hospital. The request will be turned over to a committee, or an organization the hospital hires for this purpose. They check on the doctor's medical school record, residency program, and references. They make certain everything is accurate and complete and that there were no disciplinary actions taken against the doctor at any of his/her training institutions.

They go to the list of requested surgical procedures (which would include things like breast enlargement, breast reduction, and liposuction) and they go back to the program where the doctor trained to make certain that all of those things were included in the training he/she received. In most hospitals, this has to be repeated every two years. On one of my re-applications, I applied for laser privileges, which wasn't a part of my surgical training program. Before approval, I had to attend a laser course and show proof of satisfactory completion.

Hospitals have quality committees that regularly review the work of their physicians and surgeons. If problems arise, they can compare the dontor's work (diagnosis, outcome, complications) to the national standards, (evidence based medicine).

One example would be a general surgeon who's doing a lot of appendectomies from the emergency room. If too many pathology reports are being returned with a diagnosis of "normal appendix", he/she will come to the attention of the quality review committee. The recommendation of the committee could be for the physician to undergo special training and additional close monitoring. Or, the committee can withdraw the privilege and deny the surgeon the right to perform that specific procedure.

Universities and Resident Clinics

Universities and teaching hospitals are absolutely essential for the training of physicians and surgeons, which means that you'll be exposed to all different stages of training, skills, and experience. If your procedure is outpatient, the paperwork can be tedious but no worse than a private hospital. If you need to stay overnight for a day or two, be patient. There are a lot of agendas in a teaching facility. Someone will come to your room and ask a lot of questions (a history) and possibly an hour later another person will do the same thing. A lot of different doctors in training will be in and out of your room. Your visits by your doctors are frequent and can be at odd hours. The final "rounds" of the day could well be at 9PM if they've had a busy day. They may talk about you right in front of you.

There are three possibilities of how you got there;

One: You've had something horrible happen to you and you came in through the emergency room. Remember whom you're dealing with and insist on knowing the plan. Don't ask the medical student.

Two: You came because of a special problem and you were referred to a specialty clinic. Chances are you'll meet a staff surgeon very early in your visit. You still need to do your homework before going to the clinic. Once you find out which staff member is your attending, check on them. If there isn't a good feel to the situation or you're in the dark about the plans, you can leave and go to a different University. There is no such thing as being blackballed. Make certain you're comfortable with the doctors and the plan.

Three: You came because you're hoping to get cosmetic surgery at a discount. Sometimes this works out well and really saves you money, and you have the satisfaction of helping to educate a resident. But, sometimes not. You still need to do all of the things I'm going to teach you in the next few chapters. Just because it's a famous Medical Center don't make the assumption that everything they do is wonderful. Trust your intuition, if you make a mistake here, it can be far more costly than going to a private surgeon in the first place. Here are a few questions to ask specific to University/Teaching discount clinics.

- What is the detailed plan?
- What is the cost of the procedure? Make certain the quoted fee includes the hospital, operating room, anesthesia, materials (like implants), and the surgical fee.
- Whose hands will be doing the actual surgery?
- Who is supervising the procedure and from where? (his/her office or the OR)
- What is the follow-up?
- What is your recourse if you're not satisfied or the procedure doesn't come out as you expected?
- What Doctor do you see if something is really wrong? (Remember, the residents have probably moved on)

Let me share with you a recent experience with one of my patients who came to me for a facelift consultation. She intended to have me do her facelift, but didn't come back for several months. She had gone to one of the university hospitals for the reduced fee which was about half of what I was charging. Unfortunately, she failed to question them about the complete charges. Although the surgical charge was reduced almost 50%, the combined hospital bill, use of the operating room, and the anesthesia bill was far in excess of what she would have been charged in the community with an experienced Plastic Surgeon. Although not common, this is a deceptive practice. I believe that Plastic Surgeons need these clinics for proper training, but the institution needs to be completely above board on what the charges will be.

It's admirable to donate your body to Medical Science,
but not while you're still using it.

I came through the system and I believe in this system. For residents to become effective surgeons, they need a place and a way to learn. Computer models are here and they can teach anatomy and decision-making. However, nothing can take the place of performing actual surgery (with supervision).

Free Standing Surgical Centers

Free Standing Surgical Centers are privately owned surgical facilities. They may be partially owned by a hospital, in partnership with physicians, or entirely owned by physicians. They have economic advantages because, unlike the hospitals, they can control the type of patients they accept. Hospitals have strict federal rules about whom they can turn away. Freestanding surgical facilities can specialize in just a few specialties such as; Plastic Surgery, Eye Surgery, or Orthopedic Surgery and they have instruments and equipment specific to those specialties. They usually won't accept emergencies or patients who aren't in good health. They stock only what is necessary for the specialties working there. With their economy of focus they can offer good rates for the patients utilizing those facilities, and without emergencies, the schedule runs more predictably.

They have to go through a credentialing process just like a hospital. The two most common credentialing agencies are JCAHO[A], or Quad A[A]. Most states and the Feds require certification for an outpatient facility offering general anesthesia. Be careful, I didn't say ALL states. If you're going to have surgery in a free standing surgical facility, it's prudent to check on their certification, which you can do online (see appendix).

Scheduling

To avoid frustration, It's helpful to understand how scheduling works. Surgery is scheduled as the "starting case" and "to follow". That means the only surgery that will really start on time is the first one of the day. All the other cases are listed as "to follow" and are just estimates. The first spot, although usually given to children who can't go long without food or water, is advantageous. You'll get your latte sooner and be home earlier. In most facilities the first surgery will start at 7:00 or 7:30.

The surgeon tells the facility what his/her anticipated time is for doing a procedure, such as "one hour" for a breast augmentation. But, if there are problems, even minor ones, such as a little extra bleeding it may take a little longer. That surgery may take an hour and 15 minutes instead of the scheduled hour. The next surgery is delayed by 15 minutes and if something happens in that case the next one is delayed more. You get the idea. By the middle of the afternoon, cases can be on-time or an hour or more late. If you mentally prepare for this you won't be so upset. I've actually been accused of taking too long on the golf course when my case didn't start on time. If you need it, and when all the paperwork is complete, you can ask Anesthesia for something to help you relax as you wait for your surgery to begin.

Office Operating Room

Another type of surgical facility is the office operating room. Some surgeons find it advantageous to set up a surgical facility within their own office. Most states have strict regulations about how many operating rooms can be built in a given area. "Single specialty use" rooms are exempt from those regulations.

Obviously, there is a huge convenience factor in having an office facility for both the surgeon and the patient. One place to go where the paperwork has already been filled out, working with people you've already met and in a setting you're mostly familiar with.

When you're going to an office surgical facility, it is even more important to check that they have current credentialing. It's unlikely that they would be certified by JCAHO (primarily hospitals), but Quad A does certify office facilities. Some states mandate credentialing, but all conscientious surgeons will have it in place. If they're evasive when you ask about their certification, be careful. It's also a good idea to ask about the OR staff and their qualifications. You can check for yourself by using the internet addresses at the end of the book.

IMPORTANT NOTE

Some office OR's are built because that's the only way the surgeon can operate. If a foot doctor decides he wants to do liposuction, there is no conceivable way, even in Florida, that a hospital would give him/her privileges with only a two-hour course in liposuction. Dermatologists who want to do facial cosmetics, likewise, could never get hospital privileges. They're NOT even a "surgical specialty", no matter what "society" they belong to or what course they attended. They've never had surgery basic training with it's emergencies, trauma, and unexpected incidents. Practically the only way an unqualified doctor can do revenue-enhancing surgery is to build his or her own facility. Many specialties already have "minor procedure rooms" in their office. They can simply purchase the necessary equipment and begin to use it. Until they seriously injure someone, no one will know they're there. There are more of these out there than you think, Be Careful. The quickest way to find out the status of their OR is to ask; "Do you have privileges to do this procedure at the hospital?" If the answer is YES but you're still suspicious, call the hospital Medical Staff Office and verify. If the answer is NO, you could be in dangerous waters.

Anesthesia

A few years ago a colleague of mine developed appendicitis and knew he had to have surgery. Someone asked him about his choice of surgeons. His answer was interesting. He said; "I don't care about the surgeon, anyone can do that surgery. I want to make certain I get my pick of the Anesthesiologists."

The anesthesia used for a procedure has as much potential for harm as the surgery (if not more).

Types of anesthesia:

General Anesthesia: The induction of a state of unconsciousness with no awareness of pain with or without paralysis. Requires airway support.

Local Anesthesia: The injection or application of an anesthetic drug to a specific area.

Block: An injectable anesthetic agent put in the area of a nerve that targets a specific area of the body. Spinal or epidural anesthesias are blocks.

Sedation: The administration of medications to relieve fear, anxiety, and increase the tolerance of unpleasant procedures.

An Anesthesiologist is a "Board Certified" doctor specializing in the practice of anesthesia. An Anesthetist is a Registered Nurse specializing in anesthesia. In a hospital or surgical center, an anesthesiologist must supervise an anesthetist. The American Board of Anesthesia guidelines recommend that for routine cases there should be no more than four anesthetists to one anesthesiologist and, for pediatrics or more serious illnesses, that ratio should be even lower. In an office facility, you may have an anesthesiologist (Doc) or an anesthetist (RN). Ask about the credentials of the person giving anesthesia and if it's a nurse, ask who is supervising.

Smaller procedures that don't require a high level of anesthesia will frequently be done by the doctor him/herself and can include local, blocks and/ or sedation.

If you're contemplating surgery in an office facility, and the anesthesia is going to be general or sedation, here are some questions.

What type of anesthesia is planned?

Who will administer the anesthesia?

Who will be there for the recovery?

Is there an emergency plan?

Two situations that can be problematic:

1. Having the Doctor give low-level anesthesia him/herself is common. When attempting general or high level anesthesia by him/herself they are doing two jobs; both of which need to be carefully monitored. In addition to performing the surgery he/she will have to monitor your vitals (temperature, pulse, blood pressure, respirations, blood levels of gasses and your EKG), adjust the dosages of the medications, and direct the rest of the surgical team. A fair number of surgeons do this but as I've gotten older, I prefer the security of an anesthesia professional, and the freedom to fully concentrate on the case. Some drugs used for sedation with only a slight error in dosage can turn into a general anesthesia and even take away your ability to breathe on your own. (A major contributing factor in the death of Michael Jackson)

2. Some very serious problems can present in the recovery area. Who's going to be there? In a hospital or surgical center, the Anesthesiologist is required to be in attendance until the last patient has met the discharge criteria and is ready to leave. In an office OR setting, there may not be a doctor available. Even a little extra bleeding can be a simple thing if the surgeon is available but a disaster if he/she won't be available for hours.

Observations

When you first see the doctor's office, don't pay a lot of attention to the plaques on the wall. Pay attention instead to the appearance and style of the office. The colors, layout, and decorations can give you a lot of information about the doctor's artistic sense or unfortunately, it could be his/her spouse's artistic sense. It's an interesting question to ask whether the doctor decorated the office, hired a decorator, or let his/her spouse take responsibility for the décor.

Years ago, one of my "rival" Plastic Surgeons in town decorated (by himself) his office with a large fish tank and filled it with the Asian fish with giant bulging eyes. I realize there is a highly cultivated aesthetic for those fish, but several of his patients changed to my office to avoid having to look at those fish.

Take a look at the staff in the office. Do they look like people that you would want to associate with? Or, are they all walking around with monstrous breasts and Hollywood sausage lips? All of this is giving you information about the aesthetic sense, and style of the doctor

Is the staff friendly? If they're not friendly on your first visit, imagine how friendly they're going to be if you develop a problem and need to depend on them. How is the office staff dressed? How do they interact with each other? Are patients put on hold for long periods? Are there squabbles going on in the office? Is there obvious and significant strife occurring in the office? Careful observation can give you a lot of good information about the office and the practice.

If you see patients coming in who have obviously just been operated on, watch how the staff treats them. You may be only weeks away from becoming one of them.

Who is the office nurse, and what are their qualifications? Basically, there are three kinds of nurses; Registered Nurse, Licensed Practical Nurse, and some surgeons will have a Surgical Technician

The Patient Coordinator schedules the doctor and the procedures. They're usually the person who deals with the finances, insurance companies, laboratories, operative consents and all the details necessary to make your experience as smooth as possible.

A larger office will also have a billing or finance person. Most plastic surgeons also have an Esthetician trained in skin care and make-up. Their skills can be a valuable asset to the practice when dealing with skin issues, bruising, makeup and post-laser care. Some surgeons will have a formal Assistant. There is also a Receptionist, one of the most important people in the office and probably the person with the least formal medical training. The best receptionists have a friendly manner, a bubbly personality, and are meticulous about getting answers to questions and getting follow-up information back to you. When you're alone with the staff, don't be afraid to ask them about their training, jobs and responsibilities. Most are proud of their accomplishments and should be happy to discuss these with you.

Remember! All of these observations are being done under ideal conditions. The objective answers to your question and the intuitive impressions you've gathered will help you make the best decision about having surgery with this doctor and staff.

Medical Tourism

A quick note on "medical tourism", which is the term used to describe going out of the country to have surgery for a greatly reduced fee. Outside of the US, a physician has lower expenses and overhead and these savings can be passed on to you. Many foreign Plastic Surgeons are not only excellent surgeons but some have trained in Britain or the US. The clinics can be beautifully decorated, efficiently run, and properly set up for the proposed procedures.

The problem is that it's difficult to qualify these Doctors and their facilities. It's difficult to determine the exact training of the surgeon, whether he/she's kept up with their ongoing certifications or whether they just graduated. What exactly was their training? Who are their assistants and what is their training? You absolutely have to do genuine research on the doctor and the clinic if you're going to consider medical tourism. It will be time consuming and several correspondences back and forth but you can do it. You may even have to write to their embassy. You'll find out shortly why talking to former patients may not be your best research.

Surgery is not a vacation and a vacation is not surgery. Do you really want to go to some nice warm beach location, recover in your room, not even see the beach or stick your toes in the sand? They sometime suggest that you bring your family along so they can have a vacation. The concept of vacation and surgery at the same time is a faulty idea and likely neither to be a good vacation nor a good recovery.

If you're considering medical tourism, some of things you need to think about other than qualifying the facility, doctor and assistants, is the length of the recovery and how long you plan on staying there. How is your post-operative course handled? Sometimes the clinics have affiliations with a hospital where you can stay for a negotiated fee.

How are they going to handle complications? If something starts to go wrong, are they going to send you back home in hopes that you can find another doctor? What about a true emergency? Do they have adequate facilities? Are they certified for dealing with real emergencies or are they going to put you on an air ambulance and send you back to the states? (Expensive!)

If you get home and something starts to go wrong, what's going to happen? It may be difficult to find a physician that's willing to take care of a problem that occurred outside of the states. My old mentor used to tell his residents; "once you operate on a patient with complications, all those complications become yours."

One patient that I saw recently was a lady who went to Peru for a tummy tuck, all of her wounds opened up and got infected. Back in the US, she was getting antibiotics from walk-in clinics, changing the dressings herself and making little progress. Before seeing me, she had been to five Plastic Surgeons and none of them would take responsibility for her care.

Yes, it is possible to go out of the country and get excellent surgery at a fraction of the cost of American surgery, but the chances you take must be weighed carefully. Do your homework.

IMPORTANT: *Before you consider the recommendations of your friend who just had surgery out of the country, read the next chapter.*

Trust Me, I'm a Plastic Surgeon

Chapter Three
The Patients

"Let no one suppose that the words doctor and patient can disguise from the parties that they are employer and employee."
--George Bernard Shaw

Why can concealing information hurt me?

How do I know if I have "unrealistic expectations"?

Are there times in your life you should wait for surgery?

The importance of the Doctor/ Patient relationship

What are the personality types of patients?

Are there people with psychological problems that should not have surgery?

What it I'm rejected or sent for a Psychological evaluation?

Now

that you're thinking about becoming a patient, here are a few things for you to consider. When you're talking with your doctor keep your objectivity. Focus on what is said, not the "bells and whistles", the manner of speech (to you or at you), and turn your intuition up to full power. In his book "Blink" Malcolm Gladwell describes a psychologist who, after watching a video of a couple talking to each other, can predict with 95% accuracy whether they'll still be married in 15 years. Another way to look at it is imagine reading a mystery book and how you have to pay attention to all the subtle details. You never know when one of those details turns out to be important and solves the case. Bring your intuitive self and the detail observer of the mystery reader to the consultation.

When talking with the doctor be as specific as possible about your concerns. What do you want changed? Why do you want it changed? It's reasonable to mention your hope that the surgery will make a change in your life. You don't have to know the medical names of the procedures or even which specific procedure could be the best to accomplish your goals. You do need to be able to communicate your goals. I'm completely comfortable when a new patient tells me; "I just got a new job. Now I'm working with younger people and I feel like I look tired all the time." That's a classic description of someone who probably needs eyelid surgery or facial rejuvenation. Better still, if you're able, do a little research on the procedures and think of some specific question. (This book will help.)

It's important to talk some about your personal circumstances. Why, at this point in your life, are changes important to you? One type of patients I frequently see is a woman who has finished having children and wants to get some of her old body back. Now, for the first time in years, she can think about doing something for herself, independent of her children.

Sometimes, recently divorced patients have areas of insecurity they would like to address before reentering the "dating" scene. Breasts are probably the most common, either because of sagging or lost volume from breast-feeding.

Well-planned and executed Plastic Surgery can restore self-confidence and an improved body image.

It gets trickier when a divorce is ongoing and the wife wants work done on the husband's tab. I was accused by one angry husband of breaking up his marriage by making his wife too attractive. He later apologized. When a breast procedure is bundled together with another procedure to improve the tummy, marketers call this the "Mommy Makeover".

Don't Hide Anything

It is extraordinarily important not hide any medical issues either from your surgeon or Anesthesiologist. The most critical conditions would be, of course, heart disease, diabetes, smoking, living with a smoker, any problems you've had with bleeding, a history of clots, and a history of alcohol or drug abuse.

Unlike the military, where a history of drugs or alcohol in your record can jeopardize your career, in surgery it can jeopardize your health or your life.

The only death I've had in 30 years of practice (knock wood!) was on Easter Sunday over 20 years ago. I was a part of a replant team and we had a patient brought in by helicopter who passed out on railroad tracks and had both legs amputated by a train. After 16 hours of surgery putting his legs back on, his heart suddenly gave out and we couldn't bring him back. One of the team had to go to the waiting area and inform the family about how sorry we were, but the patient had expired. The patient's brother asked him if it might have been important to know that the man was just released a week earlier from the VA hospital after suffering a heart attack. His bother had made him promise not to tell anyone.

For reasons that I have never understood, many medical personnel believe that redheads are more problematic than the average patient. I don't know if they think the color of their hair gives them an explosive personality or sets them up for special medical problems. One redheaded lady came to see me after being rejected by two other Plastic Surgeons. The last one even told her that she needed to get her life "better organized" before she could have surgery. She was a hotel manager, recently divorced and wanted the confidence boost of slightly larger breasts. She was reassessing her life and decided that as a single woman, she wanted a more attractive figure. I felt she was intelligent, organized, analytical, and her goals were appropriate and attainable. We went ahead with the surgery and her result was excellent. I don't know why she was rejected two times. Maybe it was the redhead thing, but the other two Plastic Surgeons lost a good patient who over the years sent me many of her friends for surgery.

Unrealistic Expectation

Every beginning plastic surgeon is taught to watch for patients with "unrealistic expectations" that can be either obvious or subtle. Your goals may not even be possible within the bounds and skills currently available to plastic surgeons. An example of unrealistic expectations was a lady I just saw that was 50 plus pounds overweight and wanted liposuction to correct her weight problem (because diets don't work for her). Realistically, seven or eight pounds of liposuction is a big liposuction, more than that is an unrealistic expectation as well as dangerous.

Major Life Trauma

Sometimes people react to dramatic events in a healthy way and sometimes not. If a major event has happened in your life such as a death, change or loss of job, or a divorce, you should communicate this with the Plastic Surgeon. It's possible that Plastic Surgery can be a healthy part of your recovery. Remember, however, that you can be especially vulnerable to suggestions at this time and be cautious. An unscrupulous Plastic Surgeon could easily take advantage of the situation.

Personality Clash

There can be instances in which you and your surgeon just don't develop the type of communication and respect that's necessary for a good doctor patient relationship. Everyone simply doesn't get along with everyone. If I feel like I'm not relating well with a patient for whatever reason, and it's not necessarily the patient's fault, I suggest that it might be a good idea for them to consult with another Plastic Surgeon with whom they may feel more comfortable. It works both ways; if you feel you aren't relating or communicating well, consider a second consult.

Personality Types and Plastic Surgery

What follows is an incomplete list of common personality types and how people with these personality types react to Plastic Surgery. Some of these may apply to you or to your friends contemplating surgery. Appreciate who you are and use that as a basis for more meaningful communication with your doctor.

Too Trusting:

Some people are a little too trusting. "Do whatever you think, Doc," has always made me uncomfortable. They haven't committed to the planning process and a mutual surgical plan. They might be squeamish and not want to know all the details or they don't fully understand the recommendations. If you feel this happening to you, don't back off and assume somehow that it's your fault. Keep asking questions until you do understand and can develop a sense of participation. In fact, it's probably the doctor's fault. A good Plastic Surgeon will explain himself in terms that ANY patient can understand no matter what their educational and medical background. Finally, it could mean the timing isn't right and you just need to give yourself more time to consider and absorb the information you've been given. Few Plastic Surgeons charge for a consultation and none would object to a second consult after you've taken some time to think things over.

The Perfectionist:

Another type of patient, the opposite of the above, is obsessed with the details, the perfectionist. This is more challenging for the doctor because sometimes the detail-obsessed patient can never be satisfied with the results. At other times, they just really aren't comfortable until they know exactly what's going to happen at every stage of the procedure, and recovery. Once they have that information they may be accepting of the result. Sometimes they are realistic about the potential outcome and sometimes not.

As a patient, if you know you are detail oriented, you should make that point to the Doctor. You could say something along the lines of; "I appreciate that Plastic Surgery results are rarely perfect but I really would like to know all the details and steps that occur during the surgery and recovery". I like people who ask me a lot of detailed questions as long as I have the sense that ultimately they can be satisfied. It's far better to have all the questions answered early in the consultation.

On the other hand, if you really are one of those people who can't sleep in a room with a crooked picture, or have all the clothes in your closet spaced exactly the same, Plastic Surgery might not be right for you. Plastic Surgery is an Art, we (surgeons) frequently get very good results, occasionally get excellent results but rarely do we get perfect results.

The Manipulator:

This is potentially a much more dangerous circumstance. These patients give misinformation or keep changing their information. Frequently, they have either been previously rejected or worry they will be rejected for the procedure they want. Commonly, they say one thing in the waiting area to the receptionist, something else to staff, and yet another thing to the doctor. I've even had patients give the wrong name to make it more difficult to obtain their medical records. When asked why the name doesn't match their Driver's License, they say something like "I changed it". They're dangerous patients since the doctor has no way of knowing if their medical record is complete or what medical problems they are hiding. The most benevolent thing a Doctor can do for this type of patient is to confront them in a non-threatening way, review the conflicts and strongly recommend a visit with a Psychologist to help them understand their motivation. If you or a friend is one of these patients, expect to be rejected from the office when this type of personality trait is suspected.

The Indecisive Patient:

Another type of patient personality is the patient who cannot make up their mind. They have a vague idea of what they want to accomplish and when it comes down to the actual procedures, and what each procedure could accomplish, they're vague and can't make up their mind. For these types of patients, giving them a reasonable plan, allowing them time, and setting up a second consultation is usually helpful. Sometimes they pass on the information to the decision maker in their life which can result in an actual decision. They can be satisfied patients but may require a lot of extra time and some work to understand family dynamics and to identify the real decision maker. If this is your personality type, bring the person with you that you rely on to help with major decisions (husband, sister or whomever). Multiple consults are the rule and your doctor should recognize this and accommodate you. I've had patients that needed 3 or 4 years before they could comfortably make the decision.

Be careful, this personality type may be vulnerable to a strong-willed Doctor who doesn't give you any options. The plan he/she gives you may not be the right one for you but since they took the role of decision-maker, it feels right. Make absolutely sure that you are comfortable with whatever decision is made about your surgical plan.

The Shoppers:

Shoppers are another personality type that can be difficult. There's an old saying, "Never choose the cheapest parachute or the cheapest Plastic Surgeon." Sometimes these patients have been to three or four different Plastic Surgeons. It could be that they're looking for the best price, the doctor's personality, or to find a doctor who agrees with their preconceived ideas of what's best for them. One of my least favorite things to hear from a shopper is, "I've been to three other plastic surgeons, but none of them were any good and I know you are going to be the one that can give me the results that I'm really looking for." That's really scary, and sends up all sorts of red flags. I'm not anxious to accept a patient where I am the absolute salvation to a problem that no one else seems to understand. Most Plastic Surgeons don't charge for their initial consultation so we set ourselves up for shoppers. If you think you might be this personality type, consider this; no matter how much time you spend on the internet, the information you find there will never be as good as a consultation with an experienced, practicing Plastic Surgeon. If you've done your homework and you feel a connection with the doctor, that's probably the surgeon you should be working with, even if he/she is a little more expensive.

The Accommodators:

Another frustrating category of patient personality types is the accommodators. They're the people who aren't doing the procedure for themselves, they're doing it to "accommodate" someone else. They may be having their breasts made larger because that's what their husband want or another procedure because someone in their family is telling them that that's what they need. It's important to get the accommodators alone and have an honest discussion with them about what THEY really want; if anything

It can be sad when a man or woman experiencing a failing marriage comes in wanting a procedure to "save" the marriage. I gently recommend counseling, not surgery. I see one or two examples of this every year and the conversation is frequently along these lines; "I think my husband is having an affair so I thought if I got breast implants he would stay home with me."

If you're being pressured by someone to have surgery that you don't really want, find a way to talk to the Plastic Surgeon alone and explain the situation. Even if the surgery makes a difference, it's likely to be just temporary. The situation needs to be discussed with a Psychologist or counselor.

True Psychological Problems:

There are a few patients with identifiable clinical diagnoses that should not have plastic surgery. The ability to self-diagnose these conditions are rare. If you recognize them in your friends, or even in yourself, please make your first consultation with a Psychologist not a Plastic Surgeon.

Body Dysmorphic Disorder (BDD)

BDD is a mental disorder affecting 1-2% of the world's population. It is characterized by a debilitating obsession with a perceived or imagined bodily defect. From a Plastic Surgeon's point of view they represent a particularly dangerous type of patient. First, because the defect is unlikely to be repaired by the surgery and second, because they can become hostile and aggressive when the surgery doesn't produce the result they fantasized about. There have been several instances when Plastic Surgeons have been injured or killed by this type of patient. There are simple office tests that help to identify these patients. Once identified, they need to be promptly referred for psychological care. Sufferers can be recognized by an obsession with a defect that is so small it is almost impossible to even see much less fix. The second part of the syndrome is an obsession so severe that they spend hours a day in front of mirrors worrying over the defect. They are consistently late for work or appointments, and their obsession may be combined with clinical depression.

Interestingly, there is now a recognized sub-category of BDD patients that do improve with surgery. There have been some remarkable recoveries from the surgical procedures, but the referral and continuing care of a psychologist is critical.

If you're always concerned about a body defect that your friends have trouble seeing, if you are frequently late to work and appointments because you feel you can't go out and let people see this defect, if you're frequently depressed because no one understands your problem, consider setting up an appointment with a Psychologist.

Munchausen Syndrome

Munchausen patients aren't dangerous to their doctors but they may be to themselves. They create or exaggerate medical conditions to receive treatments and frequently surgery. Munchausen patients are intelligent but they believe they must have the surgery or treatment. If no doctor is willing, they exaggerate their symptoms or circumstances until they get what they believe they need. They exaggerate because they feel the medical community isn't giving them the attention they deserve and need. One danger with the Munchausen patient is that they've had so much surgery they can't be completely honest in their medical history for fear of being recognized and rejected. I doubt that someone could self-diagnose but if you know someone who fits this profile, you would be doing him or her a favor to suggest psychological counseling.

Note: *Baron Von Munchausen[A] was a famous and creative 18th century storyteller. He was an actual German nobleman who fought in the Russian wars and returned home to write a collection of outrageous tales. He was "awarded" the syndrome out of respect from the British Medical Journal. (More in the appendix)*

Rejection

You're acceptance as a patient is not a "given". You shouldn't be insulted if your physician doesn't accept you as a patient or recommends a different surgeon. There are a lot of reasons why a particular patient and surgeon/office aren't a good fit.

Below is a short list of a few things that might cause me to deny a patient surgery:

- I think another doctor would have more expertise in your problem.
- The problem is beyond the scope of Plastic Surgery.
- The possible gain from the procedure is out of proportion to the risks of the procedure.
- The patient could be unfit medically or psychologically for the procedure.
- The patient's physical condition is too poor for an extended procedure.
- The patient is a smoker who can't or won't quit.
- The Doctor/patient relationship doesn't work.

Psychological Referrals

Referrals to a psychologist or psychiatrist should not be considered an insult. It probably means you are dealing with a conscientious doctor. A brief consult with a psychologist is worth your time if you discover that your requested physical changes aren't likely to really likely to produce the changes you want. Conversely, the psychologist could completely agree with you. Sometimes the combination of plastic surgery and psychological counseling goes beyond what either could do separately. The time spent in consultation, planning, surgery, and recovery are well spent if the final results meet your goals and expectations. You might even gain an appreciation of why that's your goal.

Chapter Four
The Decision

"We need to respect the fact that it is possible to know without knowing why we know and accept that – sometimes – we're better off that way."
--Malcolm Gladwell "Blink"

"When making a decision of minor importance, I have always found it advantageous to consider all the pros and cons. In vital matters, however, such as the choice of a mate or profession, decisions should come from the unconscious, from somewhere within ourselves. In the important decisions of our personal lives we should be governed by the deep inner needs of our nature."
--Sigmund Freud

How do we make decisions?

What do I need to know before the consultation and meeting the Doctor?

What should be in a treatment plan?

How am I influenced by ads, photos and the media?

Is "Natural" good?

Scams, shams, and swindles, what are they?

What do I need to get from a consult?

Why do so many celebrities have bad Plastic Surgery?

Decisions, Decisions, Decisions

"Logical" decision-making involves assigning weighted values to each aspect of gathered information. These values represent the advantages vs. disadvantages, the risks vs. the rewards, the benefits vs. the costs. The analysis weighs all the values and the choice is made based on the highest value. Alternatively the least value choices can be serially discarded until only the "best choice" remains.

"Experiential" decision-making involves seeking out respected people who have dealt with a similar decision and asking them to elaborate their solution.

"Intuitive" decision-making is what we most often do in the real world. Most decisions are made unconsciously in our mind (or intuitively). It would be too tedious, confusing, and time consuming to analyze every aspects of each situation that occurs during the course of a day. When normal people are put into a position of making an important decision, they feel an obligation to shift into logical decision-making. They can become so involved in this that they forget that intuitive thinking is how they live their lives.

On a personal note, I discovered a technique early in my surgical career that has never failed me. Whenever I am facing a difficult surgical problem with multiple possible solutions, I read about the possible procedures, formulate plans A, B, and C and go to bed. During the night, in my unconscious mind, one of the plans emerges as the best choice. That plan has always turned out to be the best solution. Is this intuition; or is it just what happens when you eliminate the background noise from the brain. (See Appendix for more thoughts about intuition)

My recommendation for people facing a decision is first of all, "Do your homework". You really do need to check credentials, the things we've already talked about and a few more to watch out for. Then "Trust your intuition".

"Intuition is always right in at least two important ways;
It is always in response to something.
It always has your best interest at heart."
--Gavin de Becker

I highly recommend a book by Malcolm Gladwell titled, *Blink*. The concept of *Blink* is that your intuitive brain is a lot more powerful than you realize. It takes much less time to make a significant decision than most people believe. Often first impressions are accurate, but then for various reasons you mentally play with that decision until you ultimately turn it around and end up making a poor choice.

In the last ten years, of my thirty-year career, I've seen increasing numbers of patients with problems and dissatisfaction after surgery. (this is why I wrote this book). What all of these patients had in common (and what they told me) was that they intuitively knew before their surgery that it was going to go wrong. Their intuition told there was something was wrong with the office, something wrong with this physician, or something wrong with the surgical plan and yet they went ahead with their surgery. It can happen because of pressure from family and friends or just because they were too far committed to the finances, arrangements and promises. If they had listened to their intuition, they may not have had that procedure by that physician at that time and probably would have avoided the problems and the resulting dissatisfaction.

Consultation

The Consultation is one of the most important steps in the decision to have Plastic Surgery. Both from the point of "doing your homework" and from tuning up your intuitive senses. What does the consultation cost? The standard in the eastern U.S. right now, even with an "expert", is no fee for the consultation. Some practices will charge a fee but then rebate it back to you at the time of surgery.

During the consultation, it's important that you have concise goals or concerns and that you can clearly elaborate those to the physician. Your physician should listen to your goals/concerns and suggest solutions and alternatives. Remember, not all goals are possible.

The mechanics of the consult gives you the perfect opportunity to see the office, meet the staff, look at the roles of the staff, and gather impressions of the office. Don't forget to watch the other patients. You may even want to speak to some of them, although at that stage, for reasons you'll learn about in a few pages, nearly all of them will rave about the doctor and the office. It would be far more interesting and useful to ask them if anything went wrong? Or did anything unexpected occur?

Meet the Doctor

When you meet the doctor, take note of his/her appearance, style, knowledge, and how well he/she communicates with you. Make sure you are engaging in actual dialog and not just being a passive listener. Likewise, you should have a definite sense that the doctor is listening to you. The physician should be analytical and not judgmental. Make sure your doctor talks TO you and not AT you. The overall experience should be rather like meeting someone for the first time that you feel could become a friend. It's a good idea to bring somebody with you to the consultation. They can help you remember what was said and they can watch the interaction between you and the Doctor objectively.

The Treatment Plan

A treatment plan should be the end result of the consult. What is a treatment plan? Technically, it's a contract for the proposed surgery. The treatment plan includes your doctor's recommendation for:

- Type and location of the surgical incisions
- Type of anesthesia
- Description of the scars
- Level of pain and discomfort
- Estimated time required for the surgery and recovery
- Expected results
- Necessary preparation for surgery
- Amount of time off work
- Restrictions during recovery
- Things that could go wrong and their likelihood

- How complications are handled
- The possibility of a touch-up procedure, how often revisions are required and who is going to pay for that
- Alternative treatments, their advantages and disadvantages. There may not be any alternative treatments
- The overall cost of the procedure. The true cost involves multiple items so make certain all of these are discussed. These costs can vary significantly and it isn't rare that some are left out of the calculation to make the fees look more attractive:
- The surgical fee
- The fee for use of the surgical facility
- The fee for anesthesia services
- Devices, which could be implants, pain pumps, or special wound care products
- What are the extra charges if the procedure takes longer than expected (common)
- Is there a deposit and under what circumstance would it be refunded and when would it be forfeit

If some of these items are left out, Ask!

It's important that the treatment plan be adjusted to you and not a "cook book" plan. **The procedure must be fitted to the patient, not the patient fitted to the procedure**. I was recently at a breast conference where one of the supposed "ask the experts" on the panel had the same solution to every problem breast that was presented. "Take the breast implants out change to gel and put them back in partially underneath the muscle." That's fitting the patient to a procedure "he is most comfortable with" without considering the special circumstances of the patient

Caution

There are a lot of ways you can be fooled and manipulated in making your decision. Be suspicious, like grandma used to say, "If it seems too good to be true. . ."

Advertisements

Physician advertising is an area closely monitored by the ethics committee of ASPS (American Society of Plastic Surgeons). Something that is not true of some of the "alternative societies". Ads can be false and misleading. There are billboard ads in Florida for a $3,500 breast augmentation. But, what is actually included, or is that just the surgeon's fee? The cost of the facility, anesthesia and implants could be additional charges. A little like selling you a new car without the engine and being told later that the cost of the engine is extra. We all know intuitively that this is not the way business or surgery should be done.

Photography or Computer Imaging

Photographs or photo imaging on a computer are now a part of the everyday life for a Plastic Surgeon. Computer imaging for some things is so important that I refuse to do surgery without it. The most significant are probably noses; there is no universally accepted language to describe concerns about noses, and terms can easily become confusing. A word like "longer" does not really have meaning when you talk about a nose because it could be longer in any one of four different directions. It's important to put an image of your nose on the computer. You can then easily point to the image and explain what you like and what you would like changed. The surgeon can make changes on the image the same as he/she would do surgically and check with you to understand if that's what you want.

A number of patients complain that their nose is too large. What you may not realize is that a short chin can exaggerate the perception of a large nose. This nose/chin relationship is well documented and probably requires correction in about 20% of cases. Without the imager, this can be a difficult concept to explain. Using the imager, you can see immediately the change in facial balance that occurs with a chin modification. I've even refused to do a nose without the chin when I felt that the patient would never be happy with the final facial balance.

Computer imaging can be helpful with facial rejuvenation, chin and facial implants, body contouring and liposuction. It's less useful for breast surgery. The computer can distort the size and position of the nipple /areola and give a surreal appearance to the breast.

Be suspicious of good photography. We all know the fashion and movie industries manipulate photos, why wouldn't some unscrupulous Plastic Surgeons? Years ago, at a major national meeting, a world famous Plastic Surgeon got up in front of an audience of hundreds of other Plastic Surgeons and announced that he was going to present a new technique but wasn't going to reveal the technique until they had a chance to see and evaluate his photos. What followed was a series of excellent before and after pictures with dramatic changes. Momentum gathered and the audience was enthralled (not easy to do!). Finally, he told everyone that he would reveal his technique. It was all in the photography. None of patients in his photos had had any surgery, just changes in lighting and photographic technique! And, that was in the days before Photoshop. Imagine the possibilities today. The society responded by instituting rules attempting to standardize how photographs can be presented or published. The bad news, the "other" societies have no such rules.

The easiest trick, and one that I see all the time on the internet and print ads is to take the "before" photo with overhead lighting (which emphasizes all minor imperfections) and the "after" pictures with softer, front lighting which tends to minimize or even erase all these imperfections. Watch for this technique and you'll find it everywhere, even the face cream ads.

The Media

The insatiable appetite of media for the latest, greatest and newest can often lead to procedures or products being presented which are only marginally effective (if at all). Testimony of the effectiveness often involves only one person and they may be compensated by the company. Don't expect the producer of a talk show to be a scientific review committee. Their job is just what their title says, produce. They seek out interesting guests with something to say that's entertaining or will capture an audience's attention. It's up to you to question the scientific validity of what's presented. Testimony from a single person has no scientific value and is rather like the example of your grandmother who had a wart fall off after eating a lemon on the night of a full moon. Is that proof that lemons combined with full moons cure warts, I doubt it. Is the tremendous power of the media to influence people's opinion being used to educate and improve lives (our naïve assumption) or just to improve ratings and bottom lines? Distinguish between advertisements and medical educational programming. Be skeptical and remember you just might be being manipulated by some incredibly creative minds employed by the advertising industry.

The Myth of "Natural"

Another media manipulation is in the use of the word "natural", which obviously implies that since it comes from nature it must be better, healthier and desirable. If you think about the concept of "natural", you may also realize that tornados, hurricanes, poisons, plagues, droughts and cancer are all "natural". One failing toothpaste company hired a marketing expert who added the word "natural" to the brand and turned them into a highly successful company. The "natural" was in the use of chalk (diatomaceous earth) which many other toothpaste companies also use but never thought of it as a marketing strategy. Be suspicious of the term "natural". Marketers know that it lowers your level of suspicion, and they love it.

Shams, Scams, and Swindles (Let the Games Begin)

What follows are some of the ways doctors, and their office staff, can intentionally deceive you. Never forget, however, that you can also deceive yourself. Most offices and Doctors are doing their best to provide an honest and appreciated service. Sometimes, doctors might not realize that their office staff are engaging in these activities.

The Dr. Fox Effect

This name of this sham was the result of a fairly outrageous psychology experiment. A professional actor was hired and promoted as a world expert on "game theory in medical education". Several real experts in game theory worked with the actor for days so that his lecture would contain plenty of drama but no real facts. He was rehearsed rigorously so there was no chance that anything of substance could have crept into the lecture. The lecture was presented to a group of genuine game theory experts. The result was an overwhelming success. Nine out of ten people in the audience thought the lecture was informative, clear and well organized.

Even when the ruse was explained to the group, several wanted to know how they could get more information from the presenter. A presentation with little substance but with great presentation delivery is now referred to as the "Dr. Fox effect". This occurs more often in medicine than we would like to think. An excellent presentation by a good actor (or doctor) can blind you to the fact there is little substance. This could happen in a consultation and certainly could happen in a seminar.

A reporter for the LA Times once wrote: "There are implications in this study that even its instigators have not perceived. If an actor makes a better teacher, why not a better congressman, or even a better President?" Ironically, seven years later, Ronald Reagan became President of the United States.

The "Expert"

Although the "Dr. Fox effect is one form of the "expert" there are others. An expert is someone widely recognized for his or her skills, experience, judgment and character. There are genuine experts in Plastic Surgery; in fact, many. There are many more, however, who decorate their walls with plaques, magazine articles, and awards, which appear official, but all of them can be purchased. Everything from membership in Who's Who type organizations to recognition from major fashion magazines are for sale. When the salesman comes to the office with the offer of a "Best Doctor" wall plaque for only $200, why not? You are a "Best Doctor".

There is good research observing the reaction of the brain in the presence of an "expert". A group of college students while listening to a supposed "expert" turned off several regions of the brain known to be associated with decision-making. Without those sections of the brain, they were totally vulnerable to any suggestion made by the "expert". Remember the Dr. Fox Effect and keep your skepticism high. Never, ever fall for the statement from the office staff, "How could you question the Doctor's recommendation when he is a recognized expert."

Even when the mantle of "expert" is unquestionable, someone who's written dozens or even hundreds of scientific papers, who is known for brilliant and innovative thinking, and has a group of devoted students. That doesn't mean they're good surgeons. I know many "genuine experts" that aren't that good at surgery. Old adage; "Those that can, Do. Those that can't, Teach."

Confirmation Bias

Confirmation bias is the tendency to "see what you want to see", or to interpret information in a way that confirms personal preconceptions. The phrase comes from research where confirmation biases creep into the design of experiments. Many famous pieces of research have been invalidated by the discovery of a confirmation bias.

Confirmation bias can be disastrous when choosing a Plastic Surgeon and is one of the reasons you should always consider taking another objective person with you to the consult. An example of this might be the Doctor's office with an exceptionally good receptionist who is able to answer all your questions on the phone, adjusts the schedule to accommodate you, and lays the "expert" groundwork. It could also come from your neighbor or a family member who raves about a certain surgeon. You could be going to your consult with so many preconceived ideas that you miss the fact that the office is disorganized; the staff are hostile and the consult inadequate. Know and recognize the signs that you're developing a confirmation bias and beware. Stay skeptical until you prove to yourself that this is the right place to be.

Cognitive Bias (Sorry the names are so similar.)

The term cognitive bias refers to mental shortcuts or prejudices. We all have dozens of them and many are necessary to get through our daily lives. They're decisions made in the brain, which are not quite in the "rational" centers. There are literally hundreds of them and a few will have application in the decision processes of your consult.

- The Rolls Royce Phenomenon: A tendency to feel that more expensive is likely to be of better quality.

- Bandwagon Effect: The tendency to do (or believe) something because many others do.

- False-consensus Effect: The tendency to overestimate how much other people agree with you.

- Irrational Escalation: The phenomenon by which people justify increased investment in a decision based on the cumulative prior investment, despite new evidence suggesting that the decision was probably wrong.

(This is important in understanding why people stay with bad Plastic Surgeons.)

- Ostrich Effect: Ignoring an obvious (negative) situation.
- Post-purchase Rationalization: The tendency to persuade oneself through rational argument that a purchase was a good value.
- Pro-innovation Bias: The tendency to reflect a personal bias towards an invention/innovation, while often failing to identify limitations and weaknesses or address the possibility of failure. (Marketers love this one.)

Cognitive Dissonance

Bear with me for just a bit longer as I introduce you to cognitive dissonance. I feel that this may be the most dangerous mind game of them all. It can explain behavior that otherwise would be completely baffling. Cognitive Dissonance occurs when you have two cognitions (beliefs) at the same time that contradict each other. The person holding these beliefs is said to be in "psychological dissonance". This state is unpleasant and disturbing. It demands that something is done to reduce the dissonance or in psychological terms "dissonance reduction". The options include;

- Lowering the importance of one of the discordant factors.
- Adding value to one of the elements.
- Changing one of the dissonant factors.

The fox and the grapes from Aesop's Fables is one example. When the fox discovers he is unable to reach the grapes, he decides he didn't really want the grapes after all and they are probably sour anyway. The fox engaged in "dissonance reduction" thereby lowering the value of the grapes.

Another classic example is the smoker who knows he/she is at increased risk of heart disease and cancer but continues to smoke. The dissonance reduction usually has two parts. The first, is convincing themselves that they really enjoy the act of smoking (which adds value to one of the elements). The second, is convincing themselves that they're healthy and that the risks for a healthy person are minimal (which lowers the importance of one of the factors).

"The more costly a decision, in terms of time, money, effort, or inconvenience, and the more irrevocable its consequences, the greater the dissonance and the greater

the need to reduce it by overemphasizing the good things about the choice made. Therefore, when you are about to make a big purchase on an important decision – which car or computer to buy, whether to undergo plastic surgery, or whether to sign for a costly self-help program – don't ask someone who has just done it. That person will be highly motivated to convince you that it is the right thing to do. If you want advice. . ., ask someone who is still gathering information and is still open-minded.[2]"

Mistakes Were Made (But Not by Me): Why We Justify Foolish Beliefs, Bad Decisions, and Hurtful Acts by Carol Tavris and Elliot Aronson (Mar 2008)

As familiar with this as I am, one of my friends recently "got" me. He purchased an expensive coffee maker and proceeded to rave about how fantastic the coffee was from this maker and that I needed to get one for myself. Eventually I relented and bought one. It's true, it made good coffee but what he left out (dissonance) was that it was ridiculously hard to clean and maintain. What can I say, a gotcha. The dissonance was the excellent coffee versus the exceptional difficulty of maintaining the maker. The "dissonance reduction" was talking someone else into doing the same thing or "misery loves company". Before you blame anyone, realize that this rarely occurs at the conscious level. The person engaged in "dissonance reduction" just knows they feel better, but they don't really understand why.

When your friends or even family insist that you go to "their" Plastic Surgeon but you haven't been impressed with their results, beware; you may be experiencing cognitive dissonance at work. At some level, the person making the suggestion may not be fully satisfied with their result and doesn't really know why they do it but they can feel better about their decision by talking someone else into doing the same thing.

I recently saw a patient with an unsatisfactory breast augmentation, a misplaced implant and a size she never agreed to. She came to me with nothing good to say about her former surgeon, his office or her results. But, when her daughter wanted to have a breast augmentation, she sent her back to this surgeon. Cognitive dissonance at work!

Aside from cognitive dissonance, friends, relatives, well-wishers and co-workers may not be helpful for other reasons. They could be negative about your proposed surgery because you're spending money on something they can't afford. They could be worried that you're going to be too beautiful after the procedure and take their husband away. They could be worried that you're going to be looking for a new man and will abandon your old husband. Unfortunately, these things actually do happen. Think carefully about the context that your family or neighbors are discouraging or encouraging your surgery. There can be a lot more motives than the superficial ones.

Upsell and Cross-Sell

Every salesperson is trained in upsell (something more expensive) and cross sell (additional products or services). These techniques are not uncommon in the Plastic Surgery office and sometimes they can be justified and reasonable. Trust your instincts and question the surgical plan.

As we discussed, about 20% of all patients presenting with a complaint of a "large' nose will require some adjustment to the chin (technically an upsell but in fact, necessary for facial balance). Patients seeking a correction to the neck frequently fail to see the changes in the lower face. Doing a pure neck lift can exaggerate the lower facial aging and aggravate the situation. Patients desiring fat removal of the abdomen sometimes don't recognize that the skin is damaged and has lost its elasticity. A simple liposuction will only add to the problem. Is it better for the surgeon to upsell and explain these problems, or go ahead with the requested surgery knowing that you'll never be happy and need to come back for another surgery? If the upsell seems excessive, use your good judgment and consider a second opinion.

NOTE: If you go for a second opinion, don't tell the doctor the first treatment plan. Wait until they offer their own. The reaction of the second doctor, the comparison of the two plans, and the doctor's reaction to the first plan can be very informative.

I recently had a patient come to my office with the complaint that one of her breasts was too high after augmentation surgery. Her first Doctor had done two additional procedures to "lower" the high breast without success. She saw a second Doctor with the complaint of "too high" and that Doctor also did a procedure to "lower" the implant. She came to me with the same complaint. Immediately I knew there was something suspicious; three corrective surgeries by competent surgeons and the problem was the same? Measurements confirmed my suspicion that the problem was with the lower breast (her favorite). It had drifted down (called "bottoming out") and needed to be lifted to match the opposite breast. The problem was subtle and easily missed without careful measurements. The results, a simple surgery and a happy patient. The moral of this example; Let your second opinion Doctor work through the analysis without prejudicing him/her with previous opinions.

Don't Ever Let This Happen To You

The most insidious up-sell I've ever encountered can only occur in an office operating room. Hospitals and freestanding centers would never permit it. It's a devious combination of up-sell, cross-sell, and double bind. The game is played as follows, but be aware that there can be variations. After your consultation, surgical plan, budget, and payment arrangements have been accomplished, the day of the surgery arrives. Obviously anxious, you change to the OR garb and are ready to go back to the operating room. Just before you go back, a nurse or "patient coordinator" comes up to you and says; "I just talked to Dr. _____ and he thinks that you would get a better result if he could do a neck lift, and a little tightening of your eyelids." (or the equivalent)

Now you are in a bind because you've just been told that the doctor thinks he really needs to do these extra procedures. If you don't agree and the results are unsatisfactory, they will be YOUR fault. If you do agree, these are procedures you haven't researched, prepared for, warned your family about, or planned for in your budget, (which could cost additional thousands of dollars.) You are already undressed, you have an IV in place, and you're ready to go into the operating room. How are you going to make an objective decision about that? Are you going to say "absolutely not", and tell the doctor that you no longer want to follow his plan, that you have a plan of your own? Or, are you going to go ahead with the additional procedures in spite of the fact that it blows your budget and there will be no Christmas gifts this year? What are you going to do?

This game is so devious that if it happened to me, I would muster all my courage and leave, admitting that it would take a monumental effort. At the very least, I would insist on talking to the doctor and asking for a full explanation of why this hadn't been previously discussed. By the way, this entire conversation and decision is ILLEGAL if you've been given any medications to relax you. This game is so insidious, I would report the circumstances to ASPS and the state.

Consultation Summary

Pre-consultation;

- Check the doctor's credentials, start with the American Board of Plastic Surgery; The American Society of Plastic Surgeons or the American Society of Aesthetic Plastic Surgeons. (Appendix has all the links.) Remember, you're taking more chances going to non-ABPS certified surgeons.

- Check on hospital privileges by calling the Medical Staff Office. You can ask the doctor's office about member societies.

- Check with the state for disciplinary actions and malpractice issues.

- Check with your primary care doctor but be cautious. They usually don't have the "eye" to appreciate your areas of concern, they're not used to discussing cosmetic problems, and they may have an attitude that Plastic Surgeons are overpaid "rock stars" of medicine.

- You can check with nurses, although I have seen nurses go to some of the worst plastic surgeons.

- Consult co-workers with caution.

- In the consultation, check the office, the staff, the look, and the overall impression.

- When you get to meet the doctor, make certain you make good eye contact, that he/she talks TO you, not DOWN TO you and listens to your concerns.

Additional Thoughts About Decisions

If you go into the consultation with a time concern (an upcoming wedding or class reunion) you're a lot more vulnerable to the games. Do Not wait until just before the event to have Plastic Surgery. Give yourself time for the procedure to heal and time to make the decision without time pressure.

How to know you're ready:

- The doctor passed your reference checks.

- The consultation involved genuine communication.

- The office, surgical facility and staff are friendly, skilled and caring

- All the appropriate safety measures are in place.
- You're aware of ALL the fees and possible overages.
- The surgical plan was customized to you and addresses your concerns
- You know the list of possible complications.
- There were no "games".

Go ahead with your decision with the confidence that you've done everything you could to reduce your risk of bad surgery.

I need to take the time to answer a "decision" question that comes up all the time. Why so much bad celebrity plastic surgery?

Bad Celebrity Plastic Surgery

Many celebrities will do whatever it takes to attract attention. They have an "attention addiction" that they can no more give up than a crack addict can give up his crack. Even bad attention is better than no attention. Drew Barrymore attempted suicide when she was 14, when questioned she said, "I didn't want to die, I just wanted more attention."

The visibility of someone with celebrity status is both a plus and a minus. We see their faces on TV, in movies, in magazines and even the grocery store check out line. They have an image to portray and maintain and as soon as normal signs of aging begin to appear, many feel they must have it corrected. From that decision, it's a short step at the Plastic Surgeon from "get me back to normal" to "lets add a little" to "if a little is good, a lot must be better". From there it's another short step to the cover of a magazine focused on "Bad Plastic Surgery".

Plastic Surgeons with celebrity clients have incredible pressure to bow to the whims of the celebrities. Their success and their livelihood depend on the continued satisfaction of their clients, even if it may be counter to their judgment. Ultimately, the celebrities are responsible for mutilating themselves and choosing "Bad Plastic Surgery" but it wouldn't hurt if some of their doctors learned to say NO.

Chapter Five
Having a Procedure

"I was going to have cosmetic surgery until I noticed the doctor's office was full of portraits by Picasso."
--Rita Rudner

"You only live once, but if you do it right, once is enough."
--Mae West

Is there one way to do a procedure that gives the best results?

Is it OK to ask for special treatment?

What happens in the pre-operative office visit?

What things can I do to prepare?

What happens in the pre-op area, the OR and the post-op recovery?

What do I expect when I get back home?

Many Roads Lead to Rome

Before getting involved in the details of particular procedures, there are a few things to think about. Excellence in cosmetic surgery occurs because of two things, the skill of the surgeon and the frequency that he/she performs the procedure. There are probably 15 different ways to do a face-lift. Some techniques have been developed in the last 10 years that could be considered the "latest and greatest". A good Plastic Surgeon will obtain excellence with the technique he is accustomed to and has spent years refining; not necessarily the "latest and greatest".

The frequency of a particular procedure will also have a direct correlation to how effective the procedure is and how often problems occur. As an example, nationally reported data showed a wide discrepancy in the complication rate (including death) of coronary bypass surgery from one hospital to another. Investigators were compelled to look deeper and try to discover the cause. The difference was in how often the procedure was performed. The hospital systems that had dozens of bypasses weekly had complication rates in the low single digits while equally good hospitals with only one or two bypasses a month had rates well into double digits.

This is just as true of Plastic Surgery. The variety of procedures in Plastic Surgery means that few surgeons will have dozens of the same case every week. The frequency and experience of the surgeon is still the best determinant of excellence in the result. Remember to ask your surgeon how often they perform your procedure. When I was a member of a five-man group, we made a list of problems we rarely saw, maybe once or twice a month and asked each member of the group if they were especially interested in those problems. We took the list to our scheduling people and had the patients routed to the Doctor who was the most interested. That allowed the Doctor to keep up his skills without trying to split them among five Doctors.

Don't Be Special

Surgeons have a "groove"; a flow, and a rhythm of their surgery which keeps them focused and at peak performance. The "groove" is different from one surgeon to another but we all have them. When you ask or expect to be treated "special" you risk disrupting the "groove" which can lead to an increased risk of complications.

Many years ago, one of the pioneers of coronary bypass surgery began having chest pains. He was published extensively, well recognized and had run numerous courses teaching the technique to other surgeons. When his cardiac catheterization showed blockages, which could only be corrected by his technique, he began to grow long hair and a beard. With his new look and a false name he went to surgery with one of his most promising students. The surgery was flawless and in the recovery room he disclosed his actual identity. Why? He was convinced that if he was treated "special" he was far more likely to have problems. Enough said!

Your Pre-operative Office Visit

Most states require that you have a final office visit about a week prior to the actual surgery. This is a good opportunity to discuss any last-minute concerns you have. Be certain you know the surgical plan, the postoperative restrictions, and the period of recovery. Laboratory tests, x-rays, EKGs, mammograms and financial arrangements are all finalized at this time. If you haven't already arranged them, the post-operative appointments will be made. Any medical clearances or letters from your other doctors must be on the chart or on the way by now. Prescriptions are usually given out with their explanations so they can be filled and waiting when you return home. Bandage or drain instructions will be discussed now and again in the postoperative area.

Getting Ready

1. **Reduce or eliminate blood thinners:**
    a. Stop Aspirin – you may need to discuss this with your primary care or cardiologist if they prescribed it. Aspirin interferes with the function of the platelets and reduces your ability to clot and stop bleeding. Aspirin is much longer acting than most people realize and should be stopped

2 to 3 weeks prior to a procedure. Even the mini aspirin will interfere with clotting.

b. If you're on a prescription blood thinner you must have a plan to temporarily reduce the dosage or reverse it.

c. Liquid vitamins (Vitamin C, fish oil, flax oil, etc.) are mild blood thinners and should be discontinued 1-2 days before the surgery.

2. Stop smoking:

Smoking is the most preventable source of complications in Plastic Surgery. Increasingly, conscientious Plastic Surgeons are refusing surgery for smokers. Smoking causes the small blood vessels of the skin to constrict, reducing the blood supply. During a facelift, and many other procedures, areas of thin and fragile skin, such as the neck can be irreparably damaged. The result of smoking after a facelift can be a major loss of skin, scarring, and the need for multiple corrective surgeries. I've even had patients develop problems from living with a smoker. **Never** allow someone to smoke in your car or allow yourself to be in a tight-closed environment with a smoker.

Any doctor who will do a facelift on a smoker is suspect and should be avoided. In my office I make patients promise to quit three weeks before a facelift procedure. The day prior to the surgery, we do a urine test to see if they have kept their word. If the test is positive for smoking byproducts we cancel their case.

It used to be that only facelifts, skin grafts and flaps required the patient to quit smoking. As more evidence accumulates, some Plastic Surgeons won't do any major procedure on smokers. I would expect that trend to continue.

Picture a malpractice attorney, "Doctor, you were fully aware that smoking increased the risk of this problem, yet you went ahead with the surgery anyway. Why is that, Doctor?" In England they studied workers with fractured legs and discovered that the return to work for a non-smoker was three months but for a smoker it was six months. Who knew?

3. Herbal supplements are REAL medications.

Most people consider herbal medications as nutritional supplements since they don't require a prescription. They forget that they can have powerful effects and conflicts with other medications. Even though it may be embarrassing to present a complete list of herbal meds to your doctor, do it. He probably has his own list. Also, make certain you tell your anesthesiologist.

4. Alcohol

Consuming more than a glass of wine the night before surgery has been shown to increase bleeding and bruising. Drinking after surgery, if you're on narcotic pain meds, is dangerous and the combination has been responsible for many deaths.

5. Do not stop essential medicines

Thyroid, cardiac, anti-depression, blood pressure meds and some others cannot be stopped without discussing with your doctors. They may even need to be taken on the day of surgery with a tiny sip of water.

Insulin and diabetic meds need to have a plan to adjust the dosage before the surgery and in the recovery period.

6. Some supplements that may enhance healing:

a. Vitamin C is a cofactor in healing and I usually suggest beginning some extra C a week prior to the surgery and continuing through the healing period.

b. Multivitamins twice a day. At any given time, 40% of the US is on a diet and many others are probably not getting a full complement of vitamins and minerals. A double dose of inexpensive multivitamins is cheap insurance.

c. Homeopathic and herbal aids.

d. Arnica – is a homeopathic medication, shown to reduce bruising in the post-operative period. Moderately effective now but experiments with high dose arnica (not yet FDA approved) show dramatic promise. Read the directions carefully and don't touch the tablets or it doesn't work. Arnica also comes in an ointment but it shouldn't be used near cuts or wounds.

    e. Bromelian, 500 mg. three times a day, is derived from pineapple and other fruits, and may help the swelling resolve faster.

7. You will probably get instruction from the doctor's office to take your shower the night before surgery. They may even give you some special soap to use. If the area of your surgery is hairy, **DO NOT** shave yourself. Shaving more than a few hours before surgery actually increases the risk of infection. Any shaving needs to be done will be done by the OR staff at the time of surgery.

8. Your clothing should be easy to get on and off and please don't bring money or jewelry to the surgical facility. Why take a chance? Make certain you have a proper ride to and from the surgical facility. It's probably not a good idea to bring the heavy-duty truck unless that's all you have. A bouncy ride back home can be uncomfortable. In most states it's illegal to be picked up by a cab.

9. Plan for nausea: You may want to have something in the car just in case it comes on faster than you expected. At home, have some ginger ale, soda crackers or, my personal favorite, grating a small amount of ginger root in a cup of mild black tea.

Even Smart people do dumb things!

A hospital nurse scheduled for breast reconstruction was on a powerful beta-blocker medication to control her blood pressure. Realizing that after surgery she probably wouldn't feel well for a few days, she went ahead and took 4 days worth of her medication without telling anyone. During the induction (the start of anesthesia) her heart stopped. We did CPR, she responded and was admitted to the intensive care unit for several days. She recovered well with only a sore chest. She sent me Christmas cards for years but I still think she is at least partially responsible for my hair loss.

At the Surgical Facility

Most moderate to large surgical facilities are divided into three distinct areas, each run by nurses with special training for their particular area. They are the pre-op area, the operating room, and the post-op or recovery area (PACU).

Pre-Op Area

1. Most facilities will have you complete their paperwork online before you actually arrive. If not, you'll have to do it there.

2. You'll be escorted to the Pre-op area, asked to change into a gown, bag your clothes, and give your valuables to the person who accompanied you. Sometimes the gown has a heating system built in to it. Frequently, one of the nurses will put compression stockings on your legs with or without pneumatic pumps to prevent clots.

3. You will probably have an IV started in the back of your hand, and sticky EKG pads placed on your trunk somewhere.

4. An anesthesiologist will interview you. This is the time to be completely honest about alcohol and drug use (including herbal medications). If a friend brought you to the facility, you can ask them to step out for this interview. How much alcohol do you really drink on a daily or weekly basis? How often do you use non-prescription drugs? Based on your answers, the anesthesiologist is going to be making plans for your anesthesia. They also need to know about any medical conditions that have changed since your last medical history. This is the best time to bring up a tendency or a history of nausea. There are medications that can reduce (not eliminate) your chances of nausea, but they're expensive and unless you bring it up, they probably won't give them to you. If you have a lot of anxiety, and after everything is signed, you can ask the anesthesiologist for something to relax you while you're waiting.

5. Your plastic surgeon will probably come by, do a little handholding, give reassurance and meet the person who accompanied you. For many procedures he/she will need to put markings on you and perhaps make some measurements.

Operating Room

1. You will be taken on a gurney to the operating room and moved onto the table while people are scurrying around the room getting ready for your

surgery. You will likely feel cold and awkward. Anesthesia will ask you to breathe into a mask and shortly thereafter you'll be asleep. In spite of sensational stories about people that had surgery done while they were still awake, that is extremely rare. In my career I've never seen a single instance of a person that was awake during surgery. As you go to sleep, try to think about the place you most want to visit and tell yourself not to shake your head like a wet dog when you wake up. That's guaranteed to create nausea.

2. Who's in the room?

    a. Anesthetist and/or anesthesiologist. They are in charge of your sleep, drowsiness, and vital functions during the surgery. They monitor your breathing, gasses in your blood, fluids, blood pressure, heart monitor, temperature, level of anesthesia and more depending on the type of case..

    b. Scrub Nurse. They could be either a tech or a nurse. This person is already gowned and is probably busy setting up the tables and instruments necessary for your surgery. Some will introduce themselves, others not.

    c. Circulating Nurse. They are nearly always an RN who does not scrub or put on a gown. They retrieve medications, additional supplies and maintain the official record of the surgery and other paperwork for the room.

    d. Surgical assistant. They could be anything from another doctor, a PA (Physician's Assistant), a nurse or a tech. Their job is to help the surgeon. For shorter and smaller cases there may not be an assistant. Ideally, you've already met them at the office and discussed their role in the surgery.

    e. Your Plastic Surgeon.

3. Many Plastic procedures can be done with "conscious sedation" which means you'll be given some "don't give a damn" medications combined with local anesthesia to numb the area.

Note: *I've had many patients express concern about what they would say in the final moments before going to sleep. As interesting as this might be, I've never heard any secrets. Don't worry! Once, when doing emergency surgery on a CIA agent, the* *agency required another agent's presence in the room in case anything sensitive was said during the case. He was so squeamish, he stood facing the corner of the room like a punished child so he wouldn't see any blood.*

Post-Op Area (Recovery or PACU)

1. You'll gradually (or sometimes suddenly) wake up in the care of a new group of nurses specializing in recovery.

2. It's a good idea to familiarize yourself with the standard non-verbal pain scale. (see Appendix) That way you can respond with a universally accepted number when the nurse asks you about your pain level. (One is no pain, ten is intolerable.) Frequently a drug is used for relaxation that has the side effect of interfering with short-term memory. You may not remember much of the recovery room. If you really want to remember the whole recovery experience tell your anesthesiologist and they may be able to use alternative drugs. (Why?)

3. Anesthesiologists and recovery nurses have specific criteria to determine if a patient is fit enough to be discharged from the Recovery Room (PACU). The patient must:
    *   Be able to breathe properly without assistance. (the little spring clip on one of your fingers is giving them information about the oxygen content of your blood and your breathing).
    *   Have stable vital signs (blood pressure and heart rate).
    *   Be awake and oriented.
    *   Have minimal pain and nausea.
    *   Any bleeding from the surgical site should be well controlled and minimal.
    *   On the rare occasion that you cannot meet these criteria or something unusual like an irregular heart beat develops you may instead be transferred to a hospital or admitted if you're already in one.

4. Instructions in the care of the wounds, drains or other special needs like ice compresses or elevation will be discussed and shared with your caregivers. Your medications will also be reviewed with you.

Back Home

1. After general anesthesia, it's important that someone spends the night with you. First, it's possible that you will fall back asleep and it's a good idea for someone to be there to monitor you. Second, if you need something during the night you wouldn't be able to drive to get it.

   Note: In the early days of liposuction, a group of Plastic Surgeons in California did liposuction on one of their associates and took him home to spend the night alone. In the morning they found he had expired during the night. This probably wouldn't have happened if he had someone there to keep an eye on him.

2. Remember the stockings you're wearing are to help prevent clots. Once you're home it's important for the first day to continue to move your legs. Move from one chair to another or flex your ankles regularly. After the first day you probably won't need the stockings.

3. Ice, elevation, drain care and bandages have all been discussed at you last office visit but will be reviewed.

4. You can expect blurry vision the first day from a protective ointment used by anesthesia.

5. Some leakage of blood-tinged fluid is common after liposuction and some other procedures. Most of us use a technique of swelling up the fat cells with fluid called "tumescent" and some of that fluid will leak out the first night. Don't doze off on the white sofa.

6. You should have been given a list of reasons to call the doctor. They include; bleeding, excessive swelling, uncontrolled pain, fever, wound separation, drain malfunction or difficulty with waking.

IMPORTANT NOTE

Use your good sense. If you're experiencing a symptom that would normally cause you to go to an emergency room, Get to an emergency room! Call your doctor's office on the way. Some Examples would be chest pain, difficulty breathing, hemorrhage, symptoms of stroke, or loss of consciousness.

7. Visitors in the first few days after surgery can be problematic. They interfere with your recovery and cause you to behave in ways that may make things more difficult for you. Do yourself a favor and give them "permission" not to visit you until you're up to it. It'll be better for you and they will probably be relieved.

8. Pay attention to the limitations defined in your recovery instructions from your doctor's office. EVEN IF YOU FEEL GREAT!

Trust Me, I'm a Plastic Surgeon

Chapter Six
Oh S_ _t!

"And those who were seen dancing, were thought to be crazy, by those who could not hear the music."
--Friedrich Nietzsche

"We exaggerate misfortune and happiness alike. We are never as bad off or as happy as we say we are."
--Honore de Balzac

Why patients can be dissatisfied with their surgery?

What are some of the common annoyances or complications?

What else can make for an unhappy patient?

What are some of the scams, shams, and swindles that offices and Doctors can use?

When do I need a second opinion and how do I do that?

When does "dissatisfied" become "malpractice"?

The Dissatisfied Patient

As I have previously said, nearly every patient that I've seen with a problem or a complication after surgery knew during their consultation that their surgery wasn't going to go well but went ahead with the procedure anyway. Is this a failure of the consultation process? YES!

The four main causes of dissatisfaction:

1. Poor patient selection. (See Chapter 3)
2. Patient expectations were not met.
   a. Unanticipated complications – pain, swelling, bruising, hair loss, drains
   b. Unstated and/or unrealistic goals
   b. Unrealistic timetable - return to work, disability
   c. Unnoticed imperfections emphasized by the surgery
   d. Failure of the anticipated social reaction - lack of support, empathy
3. Outside pressures caused them to question the results.
4. Something actually went wrong.
   a. Surgical error
   b. Patient error
   c. Random error

Poor Patient Selection

This is a topic we've dealt with on several levels. The patient with true pathology, the patient who has psychological or physical issues which can never be satisfied, and the patient who is unable or unwilling to establish meaningful communication with a trusting doctor/patient relationship should not have surgery. If they did have surgery and now are unsatisfied, this is a failure of the consultation process and the surgeon who performed the procedure. If they (or you) had misgivings about the surgery but went ahead and now feel it was a mistake, explain this to the surgeon but start looking for a second opinion doctor.

Patient Expectations Not Met

Keeping the lines of communication open, good discussions with the doctor and time will cure many of these issues. In spite of extensive pre-operative discussions of the potential problems, the patient may still be sometimes caught "off guard" and the overall experience jeopardized. It's always a possibility that the Doctor believed his own marketing and "overpromised" or promised more than the procedure can deliver. It may require a second opinion to determine if the procedure was inadequately done or too much expectation was placed on it.

'The chances of a complication may only be 1%
but if you're the one it happens to
the chances are 100%."
---Surgical Saying

Complications (Annoyances Level 1)

We're going to review the serious (Level 2 and 3) complications in the chapters outlining the specific procedures. Even the Level 1 annoyances can lead to an unsatisfied patients if they are more than you expected or persist longer than anticipated.

Pain: All doctors try to estimate a patient's pain tolerance, their history with painful stimuli, prepare them for their upcoming surgery, and medicate them appropriately. There are so many variables that dosage and choice of medication errors are not rare. Fortunately, these errors can usually be corrected with adjusting the dosage or writing another prescription.

Swelling: The amount and duration of postoperative swelling can be disturbing to the recovering patient and can difficult to predict. I've seen swelling of the face take three months to finally resolve and I've had others, which resolved in a matter of days. Ice, elevation and time are the main tools to help with swelling.

Bruising: Eliminating blood thinners prior to the surgery reduces but doesn't eliminate the risk of bruising. It can still occur and be distressing if you are not prepared for it. Bruises resolve differently for different patients and in different areas of the body. On the face, most bruising will resolve (after some dramatic color changes) in 10-12 days. Double or triple that time for bruises of the legs or body.

Hair Loss: Minor hair loss is common when operating in or near hair bearing areas. The hair follicles are sometimes "shocked" by the surgery causing a temporary loss of hair. The affected area is usually small and the hair will return in a few weeks.

Drains

Procedures requiring a drain can take longer for safe removal than anticipated. Not only does this require extra (unplanned) office visits but the drains can become uncomfortable or painful.

Unstated or Unrealistic Goals

Even after consultation, formation of the surgical plan, imaging on the computer, and photographic analysis, some patients will still have a fantasy idea of the final result. This has improved with the wide spread use of computer imaging, but there are areas that are poorly represented by the computer such as breast surgery. Ask your doctor to show you the changes on the computer as many times as you need. You can also look through their photo albums. Realize that these photos are probably his/her "best ever" patients. Most doctors don't want to give you a printed copy of your imaging for legal reasons.

Unrealistic Timetable

Most patients have watched some Reality TV shows where the time from consultation to full recovery takes less than an hour and the time to the beautiful end result appears to take only days. Of course we all know this isn't the real world but these shows have an effect, if only subconsciously. Although some are surprised at how fast and easy the recovery is, others will be disappointed. A patient recovering from a facelift can go back in public in about 2 weeks, breast augmentation a few days, liposuction patients are up and moving in a few days but the final results can take 3 to 6 months to see. If you have an upcoming important event, make certain the Doctor knows about it.

When patients ask me, "How long does it take to heal?" there are at least four answers;

- The time to remove any sutures, drains and steri's.
- The time to return to work.
- The time to resume sports activities.
- The time of final healing with mature scars (1 year minimum).

Unnoticed Imperfections

Thank heavens for photographs. Complaints of post-operative imperfections is a frequent occurrence in Plastic Surgery and a primary source of "Hey Docs". "Hey Doc" how come my smile is now crooked? "Hey Doc" my one eyebrow is lower. "Hey Doc" I have a dent in my hip after the lipo. "Hey Doc" how come I have a groove on one side of my face? Time to get out the pre-operative photos and show them that most of this was present before the surgery.

Believe it or not, humans aren't symmetrical. When the fertilized cell divides for the first time, the two cells don't perfectly match up and there is always an asymmetry. Look carefully in the mirror, you may notice that one corner of your mouth is higher, likewise your eyes and eyebrows. If you construct two photographs, one made only from the right side of your face and one made only from the left, not only are they not identical, sometimes they barely look like relatives.

Literally, dozens of times a year we have to bring up photos of the (sometimes angry or upset) patients and show them that the asymmetry was always there. Of course it would have been better to point these defects out before surgery.

Failure of the anticipated social reaction

Hairdressers, photographers, artists and Plastic Surgeons are some of the people who've trained themselves to continue to "see" details when they look at another person. For the most part, the rest of the population "looks, but doesn't see". I, like all of you, have experienced this first hand. Like the time I cut off my beard of many years and my children didn't notice for two weeks. A patient who has just had their nose completely redone with an excellent result can be distressed when one of their close friends asks them if they have a new hairstyle. Conversely, one of my patients, wanting to disguise her new breasts at a family reunion, had a young cousin stand up at the dinner table and announce, "You've got new boobies." (This may have been avoided with a different wardrobe choice.)

Outside Pressures Cause Them to Question the Results

Families and spouses who were not entirely in favor of the surgical procedure or who weren't involved in the planning, may become insensitive and even cruel. One husband turned vicious and completely unsupportive after his wife's self-financed breast surgery. Weeks later he admitted he was hoping she was going to give him that money for a new hunting truck. If you're receiving outside pressures in spite of a good result, sometimes it's good to discuss these with the doctor or an outside counselor.

These situations are, unfortunately, too common. Your friend or neighbor criticizes your result to the point that you begin to believe that something is, in fact, wrong.

Some potential reasons:

- Your neighbor never visualized and understood the original problem and can't appreciate the improvement.
- They're jealous of the result because they worry you're too attractive, will take their husband, or can't afford it themselves.
- They were left out of the planning and decision and are now resentful.

These situations are so common, you just have to prepare yourself for them and plan your approach to dealing with them. Many people just choose to hide their surgery and not tell anyone. Others, with more supportive spouses/families and friends involve them early on and recruit them into being supportive (best option).

A situation that I face frequently occurs in the operating room. I bring a patient to the OR for a procedure. OR protocol dictates that while the patient is still awake in the OR, the talking and commotion is kept to a minimum. Once the patient is asleep, one of the nurses or anesthesia personnel will comment something like, "She looks just fine, I don't think she needs to have anything done." My comments go something like, "First, you're seeing her laying down which, unless you're a hooker, is not the way she lives her life (Most problems are reduced when lying down.) Second, you haven't spent an hour or more talking with her trying to understand what concerns her. Third, you don't understand the surgical plan and what I can accomplish." After the procedure they always say, "Now I see a big difference, much better". If that happens with surgical personnel, you can see why it's easy for your neighbor to be insensitive even if it's unintentional.

Something Went Wrong

A "Complication" is an unanticipated problem that arises following, and is a result of, a procedure, treatment, or illness. A complication is so named because it complicates the situation. It can jeopardize the expected outcome and subsequent wellbeing. That's one official definition. It's an imprecise term since it can refer to anything from a minor inconvenience to an irreparable catastrophe. For the purpose of this book and to help you better understand the possibilities, I will separate "complication" into 3 categories:

- "Inconvenience" or level 1
- "Difficulty" or level 2
- "Problem" or level 3.

An Example: Following breast reduction surgery, one nipple-areola complex is darker and appears to have a compromised circulation. The plan could involve anything from observation, a return to the operating room, or removal of select sutures. The final result could be a complete recovery (Inconvenience), partial recovery with some color changes to the areola (Difficulty), or complete loss of the nipple-areola complex (Problem) requiring several additional surgeries.

"Something went wrong" can have three possible explanations. Although the true cause is usually a combination of them and it may never be possible to determine exactly which contributed the most. Example: A post-operative patient begins bleeding during the night.

1. Was it the fault of the surgeon who inadequately tied a bleeding vessel?
2. Was it the patient's fault who ignored the post-operative instructions, overexerted and started the bleeding?
3. Was it a random event, the clot dislodged and started the bleeding?

IMPORTANT NOTE

If the post-operative "problem" is something that you would normally go to the emergency room for, then GO. Call the office if you have time, but GO. A few examples (not a complete list) would be; shortness of breath, chest pain, pains in your calves, dizziness, inability to speak, bleeding, can't urinate, allergic reactions, wound separation, intractable vomiting and nausea, excessive swelling, or pain not controlled by your medications.

As you can see, the situation could result from the Surgeon, the patient, random, or a combination.

The first and most important step with anything that goes acutely wrong is stabilizing the situation. Frequently, the problem can be minimized with a timely and **rapid** intervention. Delay on the part of the patient, or the doctor, can exacerbate the problem. This isn't a good time to worry about disturbing the doctor's sleep and waiting until morning. If we didn't want to know about problems in the middle of the night we would have gone into Dermatology.

The bleeding must be stopped, the chest pain evaluated, tests may need to be run. Complications can be an emergency or chronic. If it's less of an emergency and you're going into the office, you need to know that the doctor is aware of the situation or better yet that he/she actually sees you. Without direct doctor involvement, the office staff are likely to give a recommendation based on the last and most similar situation; which could be entirely wrong. The doctor must be made aware of the situation in order to contribute his knowledge and experience.

Example:

Two days after a rhinoplasty a patient comes into the office complaining of fever and feeling "bad". If given the opportunity, the doctor can sort this out, treat, or order the definitive tests. Can the office?

The possible causes include:

1. The patient's family has been passing around a "cold" and now the patient is showing the early signs.

2. Since the paperwork usually takes a few days to catch up to the chart and the office is unaware that the patient required nasal packing following the correction of a difficult septal problem. This could be the start of a serious infection (Toxic Shock Syndrome). If not recognized and treated immediately this could be fatal within hours.

3. The patient has the additional symptom, which they probably wouldn't comment on unless questioned specifically, of a runny nose, which tastes salty and a headache whenever they sit up. This could be a crack in an upper area of the nose called the "cribriform plate". The salt could be coming from a CSF leak. The Cerebrospinal Fluid (CSF) surrounds and protects the brain. A CSF leak means that the "super clean" brain is now connected to the "dirty" nose. Meningitis can rapidly follow and the next symptom could very well be a massive seizure.

Scams, Shams, and Swindles (Dr. Games Part II)

Denial

"There really isn't anything wrong." "You just don't know how to look at the problem correctly." 'It will take care of itself." All of these could actually be true, or you could be right about the problem and the doctor is hoping that you'll either accept the explanation or just go away; like my patient who came to me from halfway across the country with an infected breast implant. Her doctor claimed, "there wasn't anything wrong" and kept her on antibiotics and bandages for over a year. Use your good sense, check with your spouse or close friend, and consider a second opinion.

The worst scenario, and leading cause of malpractice suits, is abandonment by your doctor. The office staff may refuse your phone calls or keep coming up with reasons why the doctor can't see you. I hate to say it, but we see patients who have been treated like this all the time. Simply refusing to see a patient without an explanation is unacceptable both legally and ethically. There are well-defined guidelines for the discharge of a patient which involve a registered letter and offers of alternative physicians.

The Blame Game

Unfortunately, this too is common. You go to the office/doctor with a legitimate complaint of injury, asymmetry, inadequate repair, or a problem that they can't deny. They may actually admit the problem but claim that it's your fault; "You slept on it wrong." "You didn't follow directions." "You didn't ice enough." "You didn't keep it elevated." "You exercised too much." "You went back to work too early." They could even pull a double whammy on you and combine it with the "expert". It has to be your fault; our doctor is the world famous expert in this surgery and couldn't possibly make that kind of mistake. They could be right, but you have you post-operative instructions that you followed.

If you resumed smoking, it probably IS your fault.

Even if you are responsible for the problem, the office/doctor is still obligated to help you get the best possible solution.

The Billy Crystal Office (Mahvelous Dahling)

Named for a skit and later a song by Billy Crystal. Some office staff barrage you with how good you look at every visit. ("You look Mahvelous Dahling.") Everyone in the office complements your new look each time you go to the office. If you hear that repeated enough times you assume they know better than you and there really isn't anything wrong. If you're convinced there is something wrong, confront the Doctor and ask directly. The office may really be saying, "you look great (for this stage of your surgery)". Ask them what they mean.

Second Opinions

When and how do you get a second opinion? Senior Plastic Surgeons who've been witness to a steady increase in the number of patients needing help or repair all agree that most patients stayed too long with their original surgeon. In my practice, these patients now represent over 20% of my total practice

Realize that bad things happen to good doctors and what happens after surgery if something goes wrong determines how good your doctor really is. No matter how expert, in the genuine sense of expert, or how skilled the physician, there are going to be random events that occur that will not deliver the result that neither you nor the doctor wants.

> *"The only way to have NO complications is to NOT operate."*
> *--Surgical Saying*

Frequently when things are going wrong and decisions are required, you can be overwhelmed. A seemingly simple correction from an authority figure (the Doctor) has a lot of appeal, even though the intuitive part of your brain is screaming "enough is enough!" People have no real reference for what the appropriate point is to make a change and that is another one of the reason I wrote this book. So when your doctor tells you "one more time and we'll have it fixed". It can be a difficult decision to make.

I've consulted on patients who stayed with their original surgeon five or more years, with ten or more surgeries and additional expenses of tens of thousands of dollars and they still did not have an acceptable result.

IMPORTANT NOTE

TWO (not three) Strikes and You're Out

I don't mean that you have to abandon your original doctor but after one failed attempt to correct your problem, you seriously need to consider getting a second opinion. You should be able to discuss this with your doctor in a meaningful way. After all, the surgery is about you, getting you what you want, and what you were told you would get. It's not about your doctor's ego. If you feel that you can't discuss it with your doctor, your decision is made.

Reasons Your Doctor May Not Be Happy About a Second Opinion

Your doctor may be concerned that since an error was made, a second opinion will expose the error to criticism. He/she might also be concerned that a second opinion would increase the likelihood of a malpractice suit; when, in fact, the opposite is true. Studies have shown that most patients don't sue because of an error but rather because of a break down in communications with the doctor and a denial of the problem.

They may resent the apparent loss of confidence in their skills and abilities.

They might be anxious or resentful of judgment by another surgeon, especially one whom they see as less qualified or less well trained. Plastic Surgery, including the "alternative societies" is now so competitive that, not only is the training and skill of the second-opinion doctor questionable, but so is their motivation. If your second opinion begins with bashing your first doctor, you may need to revise your choice of doctors.

Why Your Doctor May Encourage a Second Opinion

A second opinion consultation with an educated, trained, and skilled surgeon doesn't need to be an adversarial event. In my practice, I offer suggestions of second opinion doctors, not because of a conspiracy but because I want to make certain that the second opinion doctor is properly qualified.

If I send a patient to a doctor who is "super-specialized" then both you and I benefit. There's a chance that I'll learn something new in terms of a solution to an unusual or difficult problem and you have the benefit of an opinion from someone who has seen the problem many times before. Sometimes it's a just a relief to get another opinion on a problem that doesn't seem to have a solution.

A second opinion can foster trust in the original doctor. By being able to put aside ego and admit that there may be someone with more experience with this problem, most patients will recognize this for what it is; a genuine concern for them and the best possible outcome.

Why You Could Be Reluctant to Seek a Second Opinion

The risk of change always seems greater than the risk of "sticking it out" and staying the course. (If you have time, read the "Monty Hall Paradox" in the Appendix.) Psychological studies on "Sunk Cost" indicate that people who have spent a significant amount of money on something (cars, house, or surgery) are going to stay with that decision as long as they can.

You may consider that seeking a second opinion could be personally embarrassing and an admission that you made a mistake by your choice of the surgery and the doctor. (Not necessarily so.) This adds fuel for anyone in your family or workplace who opposed or was jealous of the original surgery.

The apparently overwhelming task of qualifying another doctor and beginning the process all over again is daunting.

The prospect of additional charges can be a valid concern. Although I don't charge for a second opinion and a new plan, I will charge for the surgery if the patient chooses me for the corrective surgery. Even if your original doctor isn't charging you his/her fee for the correction attempts, anesthesia and OR charges can rapidly equal the cost of a corrective surgery with a different doctor. Remember that after multiple failed corrections, you may never be able to get back to your original goal.

You Could Be Refused By Your Second Opinion Doctor

Most patients who come to me for a second opinion or a problem have been turned down one or more times by other doctors. It may simply be a fear on the part of the Doctor of inheriting someone else's problems. It could also be the apparent anger and hostility you express. The second doctor can easily interpret your frustration over the loss of control as anger and hostility. When you're in that situation you've already been given a lot of bad information and had your trust violated. What you most need is someone to listen, try to analyze what went wrong, and develop a plan for correction with a realistic time table. It's likely that the plan will neither be as easy or as fast as you hoped it would be.

You've already spent a considerable sum of money and the prospect of having to spend more money for another repair can be unsettling, embarrassing, and a financial burden.

Conspiracy among doctors to cover up mistakes exists but fortunately isn't common. One famous east coast Plastic Surgeon, who apparently never had any problems or complications, was discovered to be sending his complications (some serious) out of state so that his colleagues and future patients wouldn't know.

If you're not getting any help from your first doctor in finding someone for a second opinion, your second choice doctor may be your best bet. After all, you've already done that research. When you finally choose to see another doctor, take the following with you:

a. Complete medical record

b. A copy of your operative report(s).

c. Any photographs showing your problem, progress, and especially pre-operative photos showing the original concerns.

d. Any registry cards or ID cards for implants or devices.

e. Any written correspondence with your original Doctor or office.

Malpractice

First, and possibly most important, is the fact that an unsatisfactory result does not equal malpractice. Of all the people that file medical malpractice suits in the United States, 85% will lose. Be careful of doctors or lawyers who charge excessively to review the merits of a case. You will need to use the same diligence selecting an attorney as you did when selecting a doctor.

I'm not qualified to offer ANY legal advice. I am only passing on the skeleton of the malpractice law and even that differs from state to state. Some states have mandatory arbitration panels, some have limits on damages, but all states require that the suit be filed timely. Don't expect your second opinion doctor to be your medical expert in the case. Most practicing physicians don't want to be involved in malpractice cases and very rarely in their own neighborhoods.

Patients sue their doctors for a variety of reasons but the number one reason is abandonment. Doctor insensitivity or denial of the problem combined with cutting off communications is a formula for malpractice. Other reasons can include; the desire to prevent a similar problem from occurring to someone else, to get some relief from the dissonance caused by a failed decision, or to recoup some of the unplanned financial expenses.

Two Examples:

I recently saw a young lady who had a massive loss of skin over her abdomen because her doctor injected a toxic substance under an abdominoplasty flap in an attempt to stop the drainage. Clearly this was outside the standard of care and caused the patient harm. From the patient, "I know she was just trying to do the best she (the Doctor) could." Her Doctor apologized for the problem and promised to stay with her to get it resolved. She had no interest in filing a suit in spite of the fact that this injury was going to involve multiple future surgeries and would leave permanent scars on her abdomen.

The second example was a lady with a relatively modest rhinoplasty. After nasal surgery, the tip of her nose would turn a distressing blue color whenever she was in the cold. She was adamant that she was going to sue because her doctor wouldn't acknowledge that there was a problem and wouldn't offer any plan to correct it. Fortunately, the problem corrected itself while she was in preparation for the suit.

The Necessary Elements of a Malpractice Case:

- A doctor-patient relationship existed (not a chat at a cocktail party).
- The doctor caused harm in a way that a competent doctor under the same circumstances would not have, or the treatment was "outside the standard of care" (This requires an expert.).
- The injury led to specific damages such as physical pain, mental anguish, additional medical bills, or lost work and earnings.
- The injury can be assigned a dollar value.

Some of the more common claims include; failure to diagnose, improper treatment, or failure to warn about known risks (informed consent). The disclosure of risks can be difficult to interpret since the law doesn't require that All known risks are disclosed.

Finding an appropriate expert is not always simple. The ASPS has set strict rules about being an "expert" and a member who violates these rules is subject to suspension or sanction. The rules are not to protect the doctors but rather to insure that any physician who claims to be an expert is in fact a genuine expert on that problem.

Most malpractice insurance carriers give the doctor the final decision on proceeding with a trial or making a settlement out of court. Unless you're trying to be punitive, a settlement could be a good alternative. Some conscientious doctors will offer a full or partial refund, independent of the malpractice carrier, to help in the event of a problem, even though there is little likelihood of a successful suit. It's not a bad idea to discuss the possibility of a refund with your doctor, especially if the problem has caused you to miss work or have costly additional expenses.

Once you threaten a malpractice action, most malpractice carriers require that the doctor/patient relationship terminates and any further communication is conducted through the attorneys.

Part II
Introduction

The second part of the book will introduce you to the Plastic Surgery procedures in detail with a template that gives convenient and useful information about them. To review all possible complications for all surgeries is not possible. Here, we'll review the most common complications, provide suggestions for treatment and indicate what can and cannot be treated. Most of these situations should be discussed with your doctor.

Complications in General

Bleeding

Bleeding is common in all surgeries and can be diffuse, localized, or ongoing. If the bleeding is leaking into the drains or the bandages, you can estimate the amount. You should have been given guidelines of how much bleeding is reasonable for your procedure. If the bleeding seems excessive and you can't reach your Doctor's office, you need to be seen in an Emergency Room.

Significant bleeding under the skin may not show on the bandages and may just look like dark colored swelling. This type of bleeding (hematoma) is dangerous because the true volume can be hidden and it can pressure in the tissues can build up causing the circulation to the area to be compromised. Untreated, this can lead to damage of the overlying skin. (A major concern with facelifts) Bleeding can also indicate that there has been some disruption or damage to the surgical site itself and require a repair.

Swelling

Swelling will occur in almost any procedure, but when the swelling is significant enough that it begins to jeopardize the circulation to the tissues, then it becomes a significant issue. This can require a trip to the office or the emergency room. Sometimes, it can be difficult to tell if the problem is swelling or bleeding. If the swelling begins to cause numbness or disrupts function it is more serious. The most common way of preventing swelling is by keeping the area elevated (if possible) and the use of ice compresses. Some reference to these should be in your post-operative instructions.

Scarring

All surgical incisions will result in a scar. The role of the Plastic Surgeon is to handle the tissues in ways that minimize scarring and be the least visible. Things that impact scar quality can be: the type of suture, the type of closure, the location, the placement and angle of the incision, and the follow-up treatment. Compounding problems such as infection, wound separation, or surgery in areas of the body that are difficult to surgically clean, all can contribute to scar quality. There are also ethnic variations in scaring. (Asian and African skin have more problems than Irish or Northern European.)

Keloids are poorly understood even by other doctors. When is a scar a keloid, verses a hypertrophic scar? Every raised and bumped up scar is not necessarily a keloid. A keloid is a true disease at the cellular level of the body. Under normal circumstance, a chemical signal is released as wound healing nears completion. This signal turns off the cells responsible for the healing process. People who are prone to keloids have a defect in this chemical messenger system and the healing process doesn't stop. By definition, a keloid is a scar, which "exceeds the bounds of the original injury". Keloids can be very difficult to treat but sometimes they can be avoided. Keloid formers should NOT have their ears pierced. Asians and Africans have the highest rate of keloids. At some point during a consultation, your doctor will probably ask you if you have any bad scars (to check if you are a keloid former). If no one asks and you have bad scars, offer to show them.

A hypertrophic scar is just a medical name for a bad scar. It could have been caused because it's in a bad location, an infection set in before the scar was completely healed or even that the wound was never repaired. What appears to be a minor cut, if not properly treated, can result in a hypertrophic scar.

Nerve Injuries

There are two types of nerve injuries; sensory (feeling) or motor (movement). Sensory nerve injuries result in numbness and can be temporary or permanent. A known nerve injury, such as a finger laceration with accompanying numbness, will need a microsurgical repair to restore nerve function. The distance from the injury to the affected area will determine how long the recovery will take. A temporary injury can occur when the nerve has undergone a stretch or traction injury or if a surgical current (cautery) was used in close proximity to the nerve. The temporary numbness of a facelift is predictable and will recover in several months.

Motor nerve injuries are subject to the same variables. They can occur as electrical injuries, stretch or actual laceration (requiring repair). If the source of the injury is unknown, it may be reasonable to observe the nerve injury for a short period of time while watching for signs of recovery.

The most common facial nerve injury (motor) involves a small nerve that crosses the jawbone near the corner of the mouth. Injury to this nerve causes a distorted appearance of the mouth with animated speech. While waiting for the nerve to recover, some surgeons will balance the face by placing a small amount of Botox (temporary paralysis) in the opposite side.

The plan for observing a nerve injury should have an end point. If a motor nerve has lost function, it may be reasonable to watch for signs of recovery for six or eight weeks, but not reasonable to watch for two years. Significant nerve injuries are sometimes referred to centers specializing in microsurgery.

Pain

The body's levels of endorphins, which are the body's natural morphine, regulate pain and discomfort. Those with low natural levels are considered to have "low pain thresholds" and require more medication for post-operative pain management. High levels of natural endorphins have "high pain thresholds" and require less medication. The use of the term "threshold" comes from laboratory testing of pain medications. Medicated and unmedicated rats are compared for the length of time they can tolerate their tales on a hot wire (i.e. the "threshold").

Individuals have more variability to the perception of pain and the medications than rats do. Heavy drinkers and substance abusers require much higher levels of medications. Their bodies have enhanced the enzymes that quickly break down the medications. Men generally have higher pain thresholds than women with the exception of childbirth when women are able to tolerate pain at a much higher level than men.

Medications now exist which have the ability to alter the pain threshold itself and reduce or sometimes eliminate the need for narcotics. Narcotics impair judgment, reduce reflexes, cause constipation, inhibit your desire to deep breathe and cough, and have potentially dangerous drug interactions. It's not unusual for post-operative complications to be caused more by the narcotics than the surgery. Narcotics in combination with alcohol have been the cause of numerous celebrity and non-celebrity deaths.

Ethnic variability in pain tolerance is just beginning to be explored but an overview can help understand why errors are sometimes made:

Hispanic people, in general, have a reasonable pain threshold. Culturally, however, they tend not to complain. The failure to express themselves can lead to inadequate dosages and more discomfort than necessary. Some Hispanic cultures even feel that the discomfort is a test of God and that requesting more medication is a failure of their faith. Medications are not intended to alleviate ALL pain but reduce it to the point of tolerance. Better control of pain equates to better patient satisfaction and even improved healing.

Russian, Baltic and Germans have naturally high pain thresholds and again culturally tend not to complain. With their high pain threshold, they are sometimes overmedicated when standard doses are administered.

Italians and some other "Mediterranean" groups can present special problems. The Italian population tends to have a low pain threshold, and culturally, they are expressive. That expressiveness is frequently interpreted as inadequate pain control. They tend to be over-medicated because they express themselves more than the average patient and the doctor or his assistant will react with additional or stronger pain medications. It has often been said that all of the countries that border the Mediterranean have low pain thresholds.

None of these generalities can take the place of a proper history of pain tolerance and careful observation of the patient in the post-operative period.

The Template

I worked out this template as a consistent way of evaluating the following procedures.

Who Should Have Caution or Avoid the Procedure

This includes contraindications and serious medical conditions. There are too many to list, but if you fall into one or more of these categories, you should either avoid surgery or have extensive discussions with all your treating doctors to reduce the risks (if possible):

- Recent cardiac event, stroke or TIA
- History of deep vein thrombosis or pulmonary embolism
- On chemotherapy, high dose steroids, blood thinners, or other drugs that interfere with healing or complicate anesthesia.
- Undergoing active treatment for another condition or infection

- Recent other surgery

A part of the Hippocratic Oath (although now optional in medical graduations) is "Primum non Nocere" which means "first do no harm." A class reunion, a wedding, or celebrity status, such as the mother of a rapper is not sufficient reason to suspend good surgical judgment and operate on someone who is inappropriate.

Description of a Typical Procedure

This is a generality. There may be many ways of doing something and many of them can lead to excellent results. I describe one or two of the more typical ways of performing a procedure (probably mine),

Physician's Fee

Fees are copied from the 2011 national annual survey conducted by the ASAPS (American Society of Aesthetic Plastic Surgery). Remember these are just the surgeon's fees. Not included are the cost of the facility, the cost of anesthesia and the cost of the materials and implants.

Surgical Skill Level

Some Plastic Surgery procedures take considerably longer to master than others. I've included a rough surgical skill level, scaled one to ten, which represents a combination of experience, training and special training. Remember, the best results come from surgeons and places that do the procedures most frequently.

Discomfort Level

Rated on a scale of one to ten: There are so many variables, this is a rough evaluation. Variables include; pain threshold, ethnic variations, type of anesthesia, length of the procedure, and area of the body.

Length of Procedure

Again, this is an estimate. However, if your surgeon's estimated time is substantially different, it could mean he/she is poorly organized or rarely does this procedure. Studies have been done to determine why some surgeons are faster and have fewer problems. Films were made in the operating rooms and later reviewed. Surprisingly, there were minimal differences in the speed of the surgeon's hands. What made the difference was the planning. Good surgeons like good Chess players were several moves ahead, alerting the room to what was coming next, giving them adequate time to prepare, and eliminating wasted time.

Recovery Instructions and Restrictions

All offices will provide these, specific to your procedure. A surgeon's list is shaped by his/her experience and the nuances of the procedures. My list is only for your review in the pre-planning stage to give you a general idea. After the procedure, follow their list.

Return to Work

I try to give you a general idea but it must be adjusted to personal circumstances. The return to work for a policewoman is going to be different than someone who works from home on his or her computer.

Complications (These are my definitions but useful for this book.)

Inconvenience (Level 1):

A minor situation that is common after a procedure. Inconveniences resolve themselves with little or no intervention.

Difficulty (Level 2)

This is a more serious situation. It will probably require a more aggressive intervention and a longer period of waiting. Revision surgery could be required. This may or may not be an error of the surgeon.

Problem (Level 3)

The most serious of the three and can even be life-threatening. Just like the phrase from Apollo 13, I use it to describe the most serious situation, "Houston, we have a *problem*." A problem will likely require one or more additional consultations with a new and evolving treatment plan. The problem may be completely repairable and reversible or not.

This is why you did all that homework. Not only does the doctor and his/her office need to become much more involved in your care, but you need to be kept informed of the working plan. The plan will evolve as the situation changes but you still need to be kept aware. Complete recovery may not be possible.

Example: The patient we previously discussed who had a toxic injection under her abdominal flap with the loss of a large area of skin, is a "Level 3 Problem". She will probably require several surgeries to remove the dead skin and clean the area (debridement), another surgery to borrow skin (another scar) from a different part of her body to be used as a graft. Later, she'll need even more surgery to remove the graft in stages and attempt to expand the remaining skin into a more cosmetically acceptable appearance.

NOTE for the Procedures

xxx[1] - Refers to data from the 2011 survey of American Plastic Surgeons by the ASPS

xxx[A] – Indicates there is more information available in the appendix.

xxx[G] - Indicates that this term will be found in the Glossary at the end of the book.

xxx[PSE] – Indicates a situation that is a "Possible Surgical Error"

Chapter Seven
The Skin

"The finest clothing made is a person's own skin, but, of course, society demands something more than this."
--Mark Twain

"It's a sad man my friend who's livin' in his own skin and can't stand the company."
--Bruce Springsteen

Non-surgical procedures such as Botox, fillers, peels, and abrasions still require you to exercise caution. The biggest problem with the skin procedures is that so many people claim to be experts. The explosive growth of the "non-invasive" procedures is not just because of the widespread availability, their apparent safety, and their reduced cost, but because they work. Done properly, these procedures and techniques can erase wrinkles, rejuvenate the skin, improve color and texture, restore lost volume, and complement and enhance invasive Plastic Surgery. In some cases, they may even take the place of a more complex surgical procedure. Beware, though, if done poorly they can cause permanent scarring, disfigurement and months or years of misery.

Most Plastic Surgery offices have a nurse, assistant or esthetician that performs many of these procedures. State laws vary and in some states non-physicians can even do laser treatments as long as there is physician "supervising". In northern Virginia a few years ago, a healthy young military man died having laser hair removal while the doctor who was supposed to be "within reach" was out of the country.

In a Plastic Surgery office, treatments should be part of a larger treatment plan, taking in to account your situation now, your goals, and planning for any future procedures. I consider most fillers to be an interim treatment until the timing is right for a more definitive treatment. A patient, who really needs a mini- or full facelift, but doesn't have the time or resources; can get some temporary improvement with the fillers. Even the choice of fillers is important. It would be illogical to use permanent or long lasting filler if you'll be ready for surgery within the year. For example, if you need to attend a wedding next month and would like a little "softening" of the facial lines but plan to have a facelift next year, it would not make sense to use a longer-acting filler. If you did, when the facelift is done, the filler will still be there and could interfere with the result. Areas like thinning lips or depressed scars may be excellent areas for longer acting or permanent fillers. Spas and some non-Plastic Surgery offices may offer a filler or a Botox-like agent because that's all they can do.

"If the only tool you have is a hammer,
you tend to see every problem as a nail."
--Abraham Harold Maslow

Without the ability and understanding to do a full spectrum of treatment options, there is little thought given to your actual goals. A proper treatment plan could include fillers, lasers, Botox, skin care, surgery or more; when they are best utilized, what is the most cost-effective use, and what is the timetable? The salon, spa or the doctor's office that doesn't have a full set of tools is going to fit the "patient to the treatment" instead of the "treatment to the patient".

If you just can't resist the urge to have half-price fillers or Botox done at a local spa, at least check on the person who will administer these. What's their training? How long have they been doing it? Who's going to fix it if something goes wrong? If they claim an affiliation with a doctor, how often does the doctor visit the shop? (If ever).

Even in a Plastic Surgery office, ask about who does the injections. Don't be afraid to leave, "Sorry I've changed my mind!", if the person doing the treatment has sausage lips and looks like they just stepped off the cover of "Bad Plastic Surgery Journal" They could have a radically different esthetic than you do. If a little is good, more is seldom better.

Chemical Peel

The purpose of a chemical peel is to create an injury to the surface of the skin that will recover in a predictable way. The healed result will have a more even color, a smoother surface, and sometimes a little tighter. The type of chemical, the strength of the chemicals, and the method of application all affect the final result. Stronger chemicals penetrate deeper into the skin, cause a deeper injury, take longer to heal, have more risk of complications, but give the most dramatic results. Milder chemicals treat the more superficial layers of the skin, take less time to heal, have less risk of complications and have more modest results.

There are too many different kinds of chemical peels to review comprehensively. The non-medical peels are made to be used in spas and salons without medical supervision and obviously will fall into the "Mild" category. They can have a variety of ingredients but most will have a mild acid such as aspirin (acetylsalicylic acid) or citric acid. If the esthetician follows the directions, the risks are minimal.

Medical grade peels can also have a wide variety of ingredients and combinations. Some are "Branded" such as ViPeel or Obagi's "Blue Peel". The two most common formulas both rely on strong acids; TCA (trichloroacetic acid) or Phenol (carbolic acid). Which are sometimes combined with Croton oil (a powerful plant extract). Most of the branded peels have TCA as the most active ingredient. By varying the strength and method of application of the TCA, peels from mild to very aggressive can be performed. Dr. Obagi added a blue dye to his peel to insure an even distribution and eliminate the chance of "pooling" and an uneven result.

The phenol / croton oil peel has the reputation as the most powerful of the peels. You might still encounter it, but it is now rarely because of it's tendency to bleach the skin and because it occasionally causes serious cardiac arrhythmias.

An anecdote. A famous Florida Plastic Surgeon noticed that some of his patients, although they looked good after their surgery, looked unaccountably better several months later. While being visited by a Washington DC Plastic Surgeon, they decided to investigate this. After considerable persuasion, they were finally able to get the name of a gypsy woman who was responsible. After meeting her, and assuring her they wouldn't report her, she agreed to sell them her formula. It was a phenol/croton oil mixture. After some research on their own they published the first paper on a medical chemical peel.

Chemical Peel (TCA)

Physician Fee[1] - $653

Goal of the Procedure
A controlled chemical removal of the outer layers of the skin.

Improved color, texture and surface of the skin.

Tightening of the skin with removal of fine wrinkles or scars

Alternatives

Laser resurfacing or dermabrasion

Who is a good candidate?

Patients who do not have a lot of natural skin pigmentation.

Patients with minor skin surface or skin color irregularities.

Patients with fine lines, wrinkles or sun damage.

Who should avoid?

Patients with very dark or highly pigmented skin

Patients who's skin reacts to minor trauma such as insect bites with bumps and color changes.

People sensitive to the chemicals or have a history of healing problems such as keloids.

People who are unable to avoid sun exposure in the recovery period.

Operator Skill Level (1-10) – 2,3

Discomfort (1-10) – 3,4

Anesthesia – Mild sedation or nothing. Sometimes a portable fan is all that's needed.

Length of Procedure – 30 minutes

Recovery – 3 days to 2 weeks depending on depth and type of peel.

Return to work – Dependent on public exposure and makeup skills. 3 days to several weeks.

Complications

Inconveniences (Lv 1)

Flaking, peeling or redness (the redness can persist for several weeks after the procedure, especially when working out vigorously at the gym. You may want to warn them so they don't call an ambulance.)

Difficulty (Lv 2)

Delayed healing with longer than anticipated recovery.

Areas of temporary skin bleaching

Problems (Lv 3)

Scarring from infection or excessively deep peeling[PSE].

Permanent changes in the color of the skin[PSE]

Description of a Typical Procedure

The type and depth of the peel has been determined in advance and is in your "plan." Most patients require no anesthesia and experience only a sensation of heat or mild burning. The face is cleansed and the peel painted on. Depending on the peel there are various indicators that the peel has done its job. The peel is neutralized and protective cream applied.

Recovery Instructions

Protect the skin from potential sources of infection (wipe phones, ban your neighbor's children with rashes, keep pets off your bed, clean sheets, towels and anything that touches your face.)

Cleanse and apply protective creams as directed

Avoid sun exposure, even on a long car trips. Remember, sun reflecting off snow can be as powerful as the sun on the beach.

Laser Treatments:

There are too many types of lasers to discuss them all. I will review some of the more common lasers and what they can and cannot accomplish. It's nearly impossible to get objective information from the internet. The information is either from the laser manufacturers themselves or from physicians who just spent a lot of money on a laser and need to make their laser payments.

Hair Reduction Lasers

All hair removal or hair reduction lasers require multiple treatments, and they don't work at all on light or grey hair. The laser damages or destroys the hair follicle by heating the colored bulb at the base of actively growing hairs. If the bulb doesn't contain enough pigment (grey or light hair) the procedure won't work. It takes a long time, if ever, for the body to repair the damaged hair unit. The treatments can be moderately uncomfortable depending on the size and location of the area. Sometimes a topical anesthetic can be used to "take the edge off". Treatment of a full back on a man or both legs on a woman may take several hours. The best results happen with very pale skin and darker hairs, so let your summer tan fade before going for a treatment.

Technicians do most of these procedures. You will need to check beforehand who is going to do the procedure and their skills. At a minimum, ask how many times they've done the procedure, their training, and their rate of complications. In our office, we've seen some fairly serious burns and bleached-out areas caused by poorly trained and unsupervised technicians.

Hair removal laser

Physician fee[1] - Not Available

Goal of the procedure

To reduce or eliminate unwanted hair without damage to the surrounding skin

Alternatives

Shaving, epilation or waxing all work but with a more rapid return of hair.

Who is a good candidate?

Light skin and dark hair. Grey, blonde and some red hair won't respond to the laser treatment.

Who should avoid?

People with very tan or dark skin, people with healing disorder such as keloids, and people with very low pain thresholds. People with active skin infections or a strong history of herpes.

Operator skill level (1-10) – 3,4

Discomfort (1-10) – 3,4

Anesthesia – topical or none

Length of procedure – 20 minutes for bikini area, 3-4 hours for a back

Recovery time – redness and stinging for a few days

Return to work – Same day for smaller procedures, next day for the larger areas

Potential complications

Inconveniences (Level 1) – Redness and tenderness

Difficulties (Level 2) – Swelling of the treated areas, blistering, skin loss

Problems (Level 3) – Permanent loss of pigment in the skin[PSE], scarring from deep injury or burn[PSE], systemic effects such as cardiac problems from topical anesthesia.

Description of typical procedure

You should shave the area 3-7 days before the procedure. The goal of the shaving is to reduce the amount of hair but still have enough for the technician to see the pattern and location of the target hairs. Caffeine prior to the procedure can increase your sensitivity to the discomfort of the laser. You would need to be positioned to allow best access to the area. If a topical is used it must be put on the area at least 20 minutes before beginning. A grid is marked on the treated area to minimize overlap and skipped areas. The area to be treated has a gel applied to improve the contact of the laser. The technician passes the laser over the area with sequential bursts of the beam. Some lasers have cooling built into the head others use cool air. The individual bursts are only moderately uncomfortable but very large areas like a man's back can wear on you. After the laser, the conductive gel is removed and replaced with a soothing gel. No bandages.

Recovery instructions

Avoid sun exposure, irritating clothing, and make certain the creams you have are approved or supplied by the office. Avoid activities that would cause perspiration for a few days.

Vascular Lasers

The vascular lasers have frequencies (color) that deliver their maximal energy to the blood and blood vessels. They can be used to treat birthmarks, areas of spider veins, or red marks. They can also help moderate the healing process and aid in the formation of better quality scars. Caution should be exercised when used these lasers on the larger leg veins. They could create "ghost veins" or depigmented (white) lines where the veins once were. Treatments are faster than hair reduction and less uncomfortable. Multiple treatments are the rule, but you would not need to miss work. With lasers "white is better". Let your tan fade. **Diode lasers** are a subcategory of vascular lasers with a delicate fine beam. They are especially useful for the tiny vessels around the face, cheeks and nose. The tightly focused beam allows the operator to literally trace and eliminate the "broken vessels" on the face. In fact, one of the training exercises is tracing and erasing the red roads off of street maps. They can also be used to treat "age spots" or pigmented spots of the back of your hands. They're minimally uncomfortable, fast, and don't require time off work.

Resurfacing Lasers

The resurfacing lasers are the heavyweights of the laser family. They can be Erbium, CO_2 or a mixture. Both are invisible and target water in the cells. "Ablative" treatments remove the surface of the skin, have the most dramatic results, and take the longest to heal. "Non-ablative" lasers leave the surface of the skin intact and deliver their energy to the collagen in the deeper layers of the skin, with a more modest improvement, a much more rapid recovery, but still may require multiple treatments. By removing the surface of the skin, the lasers create a controlled second-degree burn. The healing process creates a much smoother, healthier looking area with reduced lines, wrinkles or scars.

There's a fine difference between a great resurfacing by laser and a serious third degree burn with permanent scarring. For this reason, only the doctor should handle these lasers. (A legal requirement in many states) All of the cautions about keeping the skin clean, avoiding infection and sun exposure are even more important after a resurfacing procedure.

Ablative Resurfacing Laser

Physician fee[1] - $2,169

Goal of the procedure

A major resurfacing of the skin with more even color, reduced wrinkles or scars, reduction of sun damage, tighter and firmer skin.

Alternatives

Dermabrasion can do the same but in limited areas. Chemical peel.

Who is a good candidate?

Good overall health able to tolerated higher levels of anesthesia.

People who can live in a clean environment for the recovery period.

Who should avoid?

Patients with a lot of pets or whose life involves exposure to infectious agents like farming, need to carefully consider.

Patients with a history of keloid, abnormal healing, herpes infections, or patients who are on medications that interfere with healing.

Operator skill level (1-10) – 5,6

Discomfort (1-10) – 2,3

Anesthesia – General or local with sedation

Length of procedure – Less than one hour for a full face

Recovery time – 7 days minimum

Return to work – 7+ days depending upon exposure and makeup abilities

Potential complications

Inconveniences (Level 1) – Dressings, red weeping skin, burning

Difficulties (Level 2) – Slow areas of healing, prolonged redness after healing. The edges of the treatment can be very visible initially and take a long time to blend in. Allergic reactions to skin products is common after laser treatments and needs to be recognized and treated promptly.

Problems (Level 3) – Infection can spread rapidly in the laser-damaged skin, if that happens scarring will probably result. Latent viral infections like Herpes (cold sores) can be activated and anti-viral medications taken pre-treatment. Scarring[PSE], major or minor, can occur and will require additional procedures. Areas of pigment change; bleached areas are likely to be permanent, but darker (hyperpigmented) areas can be treated, and usually improve with time.

Description of typical procedure

You are brought to the surgical facility. The skin is prepared just like an invasive surgery. Anesthesia is administered either general or some type of local with sedation. The individual lasers vary but most are used on the prepared skin without additional creams. The settings and number of passes of the ablative lasers are critical. The skin of the eyelids is much thinner and more vulnerable than the cheeks or forehead and requires a much lower setting. The laser is passed over these areas with the appropriate settings until the ablation is even and consistent. Edges or the lines where the laser stops must be blended into the rest to minimize visibility. The use of dressings and creams after the laser treatment vary from one surgeon to another. Some surgeons prefer to use a type of wet-dressing, others will just use creams.

Recovery instructions

After ablative laser, the sensitivity of the skin is dramatically increased. It's possible to develop an allergy to a product you've used for many years. It's important to follow your post-op instructions carefully and do not assume you can modify it.

Visits to the office after laser are both to monitor the recovery and to help with cleaning the area. Protocols differ greatly in terms of which creams and / or dressings are used. Make certain you know this in advance and you've made arrangements for your visits. Early sun exposure can be a disaster. I usually recommend that you put a cloth over the side window when riding in a car for these visits. Most people will not want to be seen in public for the first week. I usually tell my patients, "If you cover all the mirrors, you won't have any discomfort at all."

Fraxel lasers are a dramatic variation of the resurfacing lasers. They can be CO_2 or erbium but most are a mixture of the two. The Fraxel works by laser drilling thousands of microscopic holes in the skin. The surface of the skin remains intact but as these holes heal, the procedure reduces wrinkles, and improves the texture and appearance of the skin. Many gadgets in plastic Surgery claim to "tighten" the skin, the Fraxel laser actually does. This laser has also demonstrated a remarkable ability to modify and improve thick heavy scarring. It has even been used on burn scars of the neck with dramatic improvements.

Advantages of the Fraxel laser are a quick recovery (2-3 days of redness) and it requires only local or topical anesthesia. The disadvantage is that it may require multiple treatments to get the desired result.

Pigment or tattoo removal lasers can be used to erase tattoos. Different colors of the ink require different lasers, although, some newer lasers may be able to remove multiple (not all) colors. Most of these lasers require several treatment sessions which can get expensive. The final result may be a white version (ghost) of the original tattoo. Both the lasers and the treatment protocols are improving. One recent study demonstrated that several treatments are possible on the same day with only a brief rest period. This dramatically reduces the overall treatment time and the cost.

Surgical removal is an alternative. If the tattoo is small, you could decide that a linear scar is preferable. A second alternative is to find a tattoo artist who specializes in cover-up tattoos. The name of your ex-boyfriend on your bum could be changed to a butterfly or a bat, whichever one is the most appropriate.

Intense pulsed light (IPL) is used by dermatologists and Plastic Surgeons. It uses multiple wavelengths of non-laser light to treat sun-induce changes on the face including age spots and broken blood vessels. It may even help reduce wrinkles and hair.

Since IPL's aren't a true laser, there are less restrictions on who is able to use these devices. In untrained hands, they still have the potential to cause pigment loss or even burns. It is a simple office procedure, doesn't require anesthesia, and has a very quick recovery. There is some redness and flushing of the skin immediately after treatment.

Average costs are about $600 per treatment.

Radio frequency treatment of the skin is promoted as a procedure that will tighten the surface of the skin. The procedure can be uncomfortable and many Plastic Surgeons believe that for the cost involved, the results do not justify the minimal improvements. The devices heat the collagen in the deeper layers of the skin. Collagen repair follows allegedly resulting in younger and less wrinkled skin. I've been to one major Plastic Surgery conference where the Radio Frequency devices were voted "one of the ten most useless devices of the decade". Before proceeding with this procedure, do your homework.

Needling is a very old concept that is still available, especially in other parts of the world. It uses a roller with multiple tiny projecting needles. After local anesthesia, the tool is rolled back and forth creating hundreds of tiny punctures in the scar. As the healing progresses, the scar becomes softer, flatter, and more aesthetically acceptable. Largely replaced by the high-tech Fraxel laser, the similarities are not coincidental.

Dermabrasion was originally developed in WWII when antibiotics were scarce. It was primarily used to treat acne and other skin problems including infections. The dermabrader uses a rotating fine sanding wheel or wire wheel to remove the outer surface of the skin. The skin heals with a smoother and more even surface.

Most young Plastic Surgeons no longer get much training in this technique, if any. In a few areas, such as around the lips and some types of unsatisfactory scars, dermabrasion actually has some advantages over the resurfacing lasers. With dermabrasion, healing is faster, has less redness, and a lower cost. Depigmentation, infection and scarring can still occur like the resurfacing laser. It requires a minimum of one week off of work. The dermabrasion procedure serially removes the outer layers of the skin, while the surgeon carefully watches the pattern of bleeding. The size and number of bleeding spots tell him/her how deep the dermabrasion has penetrated the skin. When the desired level has been achieved, protective dressings or ointments are applied.

A variation of dermabrasion called **Micro-dermabrasion** uses a gritty substance that is blown against the skin, a miniature version of the industrial sand-blasters you've seen cleaning old buildings. Micro-dermabrasion removes the outer layers of the skin (no bleeding) and results in a freshening of the skin. It can be done in anticipation of an upcoming social event and works best when combined with a medical-grade skin care program.

Dermaplaning is a superficial skin removal similar to the Micro-dermabrasion but done by scraping the outer surface of the skin with a scalpel or surgical blade.

Botox, Myoblock, Dysport, and Xeomin (paralytic agents):

The paralytic agents are used to temporarily paralyze small facial muscles that contribute to unwanted facial lines or wrinkles. The three most common areas treated are the forehead, the crow's feet and the glabella[G]. "Off-label[G]" usages are common and include; treatment for migraine headaches, facial muscle asymmetry after stroke or palsy, sweaty palms and underarms, painful feet, perioral wrinkles, and many others.

As you already know, muscle activity is initiated by signals carried by the motor nerves. When the nerve impulse reaches the junction of the nerve with the muscle, called a "motor end-plate". A chemical transmitter is released which activates the muscle. The paralytic agents work by irreversibly blocking the "motor end-plate". Fortunately or unfortunately, the body recognizes this and builds a new "motor-end plate" with the return of muscle activity. The time frame for the body to make a new "motor end-plate" is consistently three to four months. Increasing the dosage of the paralytic agent does not cause the effect to last longer. The goal of using these paralytic agents is to block the activity of very specific muscle units and reduce or eliminate the overlying wrinkles.

The origin of all the agents is similar. They're all derived from cultures of bacteria genetically engineered to produce the botulism toxin. In its undiluted form, botulism is one of the most serious and potentially fatal types of food poisoning. In its therapeutic form, the botulism toxin is precisely diluted and safe.

Amusing as it is in the movies or on TV, the goal of treating the sheet muscles, (forehead and crow's feet), is not to completely paralyze the muscle. A fully intact muscle is necessary for forehead wrinkles to develop. By injecting six to eight small doses of the paralytic agent into the forehead muscle you are still able to raise your eyebrows and look surprised, but, most of the wrinkles will go away. One concern when treating the forehead is lowering of the eyebrows, which can give the impression of anger or seriousness. Experience, and careful injection technique, will minimize the risk of this problem.

To treat the crow's feet area, another sheet muscle at the corner of the eyes, four or five dots on each side are all that's needed. Spots of paralyzed muscle reduce the wrinkles and still permit tight closure of the eye with protection from irritating shampoo.

The glabella[G] , an area at the top of the nose and just between the eyebrows, is a constellation of three muscles forming a triangle. Frequent use of these muscles causes the frown lines that so many of us are familiar with. The muscles can be treated with either linear or dot-type injections. These injections can occasionally cause a temporary sagging of the eyelids.

Botox injection

Physician fee[1] - $365

Goal of the procedure

To reduce or eliminate unwanted wrinkles, balance muscle irregularities, reduce excessive sweating

Alternatives

None

Who is a good candidate?

Healthy people between the ages of 18 and 65 who are interested in reducing sweat gland or muscle activity in a specific area

Who should avoid?

Women who are pregnant, patients with pre-existing nerve or muscle disease (ALS, myasthenia gravis, or Lambert-Eaton). People on blood thinners or daily aspirins are at increased risk of bruising.

Operator skill level (1-10) – 2

Discomfort (1-10) – 1,2

Anesthesia – Ice or none

Length of procedure – 2-3 minutes

Recovery time – a few minutes of redness and icing

Return to work - Immediately

Potential complications

Inconveniences (Level 1) – Bruising, dry mouth, discomfort at the injection site, tiredness, headache or neck pain

Difficulties (Level 2) – Sagging eyebrows or eyelids, double vision, blurred vision or decreased eyesight

Problems (Level 3) – Botox is rarely responsible for serious side effects. Most are exacerbations of existing muscle or breathing problems.

Description of typical procedure
A typical procedure is multiple small injections with a very tiny needle. It takes only a few minutes and is done with ice compresses to reduce the discomfort and the risk of bruising.

Recovery instructions
Aggressive physical activities should be avoided for one day. Expect the full result to take 3-7 days.

After a stroke or palsy and the weakness of the muscles on one side of the face, the muscles on the opposite side can become hyperactive. When this happens, it exaggerates the muscle imbalance and facial asymmetry. Cautiously, the muscles on the hyperactive side can be injected with tiny amounts of paralytic agent to reduce their activity and improve the facial symmetry.

Torticolis^G is a spasm, usually in children, of one of the neck muscles. This exaggerated muscle activity causes a twist and tilt of the head. It can be uncomfortable and take a long time to resolve. Botox injected into the spastic muscle can speed the recovery.

Hyperhydrosis^G is a condition of excessive sweating. When it involves the palms or soles of the feet, it can be debilitating. The definitive treatment is a major surgery but Botox injected into the affected areas can provide temporary relief.

Unusual uses of Botox are numerous and sometimes comical:

- Injections into the sole of the feet to comfortably wear higher heel shoes.
- Injections into the muscle of a submuscular breast augmentation to relax the muscle and allow the implant to position more quickly.
- Breast injections to give more lift to the breasts.
- Correction of a "gummy smile" by lowering the upper lip with injections.
- Armpit injections for models to eliminate sweating and protect the expensive clothing

One final caution. In California a group of doctors ordered a Botox-equivalent from China and used it on a patient that died from the injection. In the investigation, it was determined that they had purchased laboratory grade Botox that was intended to be diluted hundreds of times.

Fillers

"You are here to discover the subtle science and exact art of filler placement. As there is little foolish wand-waving here, many of you will hardly believe this is magic. I don't expect you will really understand the beauty of a syringe of living fat or the delicate power of millions of small beads waiting to turn back the hands of time and restore the youth and beauty of former years. Consider the power of liquids that creep through human tissues, bewitching the mind, ensnaring the senses and altering time itself."

My modification of a lecture by Severus Snape (Harry Potter and the Sorcerer's Stone)

--JK Rowling

The filler market is one of the most rapidly growing areas in all of Plastic Surgery and Dermatology. Its been estimated that a new filler is approved at a rate of about one a month. Different types of fillers, different chemical substances, duration of the fillers, complication rates, first time usage, area of use, and the mobility of the area, all affect the choice of fillers.

Fillers are natural or synthetic substances used to "fill" areas that have become deficient from aging, trauma, congenital defects, or for cosmetic enhancement. The choice of filler for the location is constantly evolving as new products reach the market. A skilled physician, able to use the full spectrum of fillers and who is well versed in the subtleties of the different fillers, is essential for a good result.

When planning on having fillers, be certain to check on who is going to do the injections; their training, experience and rate of complications. States vary in their requirements for doctor supervision. Even in the states that require it, don't be surprised if the doctor is nowhere to be seen. If your goal is a natural look, (as in human, not duck-like) and your technician has Hollywood style sausage lips, you should strongly reconsider. Their aesthetic sense is probably very different from yours. Risks, benefits, costs, durability and inconvenience are all different from one filler to another and need to be discussed in detail.

Probably the most common use of fillers is to soften or erase the lines and grooves of the face associated with aging. The "nasolabial groove" (from the corner of the nose to the angle of the mouth), the "marionette line" (from the corner of the mouth toward the jawline), the "oral commissure" (the depression at the corner of the mouth), and the "tear trough" (from the nasal corner of the eye extending at an angle down the cheek) are the most frequently treated areas.

Other filler uses include the ability to change the shape of deeper underlying facial structures such as the cheek area, nose or chin. Longer lasting or permanent fillers can sometimes take the place of implants in these areas and avoid surgery. Fillers can also be used to rejuvenate and fill out hollow areas like the temple or back of the hands.

Computer analysis and modern technology has allowed Plastic Surgeons to study the changes that take place during the aging process. One of the surprising findings was the dramatic loss of soft tissue volume in the face. We now know that restoring the volume is just as important as the lifting and redraping of the sagging skin that we've been doing for decades. It's even possible in early cases to rejuvenate the face with fillers and volume restoration alone. The addition of fillers in an area of moderate sagging will sometimes give the needed "lift" to the area without surgery. These techniques are now being referred to as the "Liquid Facelift".

PARTIAL LISTING OF COMMON FILLERS

Type	Names	Material	Costs	Uses	Duration	Cons
Collagen (Human) bovine, porcine	Cosmoderm Cosmoplast	Human or animal derived collagen	$520 $468	Anywhere	Immediate 3 months	Short duration allergies
Hyaluronic Acid	Restylane Juvaderm Perlane	Non-animal laboratory design to resist degradation	$529	Volume, Contouring	Immediate 6-18 months Enzyme removal	Cen be felt if too superficial
Calcium hydroxy-lapatite	Radiesse	Microspheres of hydroxylapatite	$626	Volume	12 months	Not lips, clumping, nodules possible
Poly-L-Lactic Acid	Sculptra New Fill	Synthetic material that stimulates collagen	$987	Volume, some fine lines	18-24 months	Multiple treatments can have lumpiness
Fat Transfer	Lipostructure	Harvested from the patient	$1,685	Volume, not fine detail	6 months to 10 years	Not fine lines, swelling can last days
Polymethyl-methacrylate	Artefill	PMMA microspheres in collagen	$995	Volume, some lines	Permanent	Multiple treatments Allergies from collagen base
Silicone	Silikon 1000	Medical grade silicone oil	n/a	Volume and fine lines contouring	Permanent	No removal, Not lips DANGER With non-medical grade silicone

Note - Many of these agents used in unapproved areas are considered "off label" along with any use of Silicone

Temporary Fillers

Collagen

Collagen was the first filler approved by the FDA over twenty years ago. The original collagen fillers were processed from bovine ligaments. Now they're human, porcine, or bovine. The advantages are lower cost, immediate effect and minimal swelling. They have several disadvantages. First, they require two skin tests to insure there are no problems with allergy. If done properly, that could mean a wait of 4-6 weeks. Second, they have poor durability, in some areas only lasting weeks to a few months. Third, they have a tendency to "clump" and become irregular. Human derived collagen was approved by the FDA and has a reduced risk of allergy, but continues to have many of the same problems. The collagen products are infrequently used now except for special circumstances. In Hollywood, when they have a need for an "overtreated look", they use collagen. It has an immediate effect, with minimal swelling and a rapid return to normal.

Names (incomplete) – Cosmoderm, Cosmoplast, Zyderm, Zyplast, Dermalogen

Hyaluronic Acid

Hyaluronic Acid fillers are very similar to a natural substance found in the skin. When Collagen proved to be such a disappointment in terms of duration, other substances were explored. One of these is hyaluronic acid. The first HA fillers were made from animal products and had allergy issues just like collagen. Now they're synthetic and referred to as "Non-animal Stabilized Hyaluronic Acid (NASHA)". The synthesized form has been chemically engineered to resist degradation and increase its longevity.

HA products have several advantages:

- There is no skin test is required for the synthetic versions.
- They have a reasonable longevity of 6-18 months depending on location.
- They are mostly free from clumping when injected properly.
- The have a reasonable cost

- They have an immediate improvement with minimal stimulation of the body's own fibrous reactions.

- They can be used in most areas of the body.

- Last, but certainly not least, they're reversible. The body has a natural enzyme which breaks down the HA in the body. This enzyme has been synthesized and is available to physicians. A single treatment can cause the HA to virtually disappear overnight. This gives the Plastic Surgeon the ability to "erase" the HA, making it the ideal substance for first time users who are not certain if they will like the effect. HA is highly recommended as a first step before a permanent for semi-permanent filler.

A partial list of the names – Restylane, Perlane, Juvaderm, Prevail Silk, Captique, Esthélis, Elevess, Hylaform

Semi-Permanent Fillers

Radiesse - Calcium Hydroxylapatite microspheres in aqueous gel.

This filler is usually injected over several sessions. It was originally approved by the FDA as a deep volume replacement, but is now used to correct deeper wrinkles and folds of the face. There is an immediate effect of volume enhancement followed by a later effect. The body reacts to the microspheres by contributing fibrous tissue and collagen that both increases the fill and adds to the longevity of 12-18 months. This filler should not be used in the lips or eyelids since there it has an increased risk of clumping and irregularity. There is no method to reverse the treatments except for surgical excision or time.

Sculptra – Lypholized Microparticles of poly-L-lactic acid

This is another semi-permanent filler first approved by the FDA as a deep volume replacement and now used in more general applications. After injection, the suspending liquid is absorbed leaving behind the PLLA particles behind. The particles induce a fibrotic response and collagen production over the following 1 to 2 months. Its normally used in two to three sessions over 1 to 2 months. Specific injection techniques include aggressive massage over 5 days and are necessary to prevent clumping and reduce the risk of nodule formation.

The duration as specified by the company is 18-24 months, but many patients report even longer residual effects. A comprehensive treatment plan must be discussed prior to injection and the filler has to be prepared several days in advance. Subsequent treatment sessions need to be planned well in advance.

Two areas that do very well with this filler are the temples and the backs of the hands. The required aggressive massage for five days reduces the risk of lumps or irregularities.

Fat injections or Lipostructure

The only "natural" substance used as a filler. The concept of removing fat from one area, purifying it and placing it in a deficient area has been a successful procedure for over 15 years. Both the harvesting techniques and the injection techniques have been refined over time to insure the maximum survival of the transplanted fat cells.

Fat can be harvested from almost any area of the body although there are a few studies that suggest fat from certain areas may have better longevity. Life expectancy of the fat is generally considered to be about 10 years. The advantages of lipostructure is that; it is a obtained from your own body, it reduces the area where the fat is harvested (such as the abdomen), it remains soft, and it's readily available in most people.

The disadvantages include; the color of the fat, which can show through thinner tissues, the natural absorption of 20% or more of the fat, the need for a donor surgical area, and the limited amount of fat that can be injected at one time. Another disadvantage relates to the "naturalness" of the fat. Future weight gains will include the transferred fat. The soft nature and predictability of the fat make it one of the best materials for lip augmentation, but be aware that a large weight gain will increase the volume of the lips (sometimes dramatically).

PERMANENT Fillers

Artefill – Polymethylmethacrylate (PMMA) spheres suspended in bovine collagen

Artefill is the first permanent filler approved by the FDA. The product is now in its fourth generation and the criticisms of the earlier types have been resolved. The material is made of symmetrical PMMA beads suspended in bovine collagen. It requires a skin test and a 4-week wait to rule out allergy.

After injection, the collagen is gradually absorbed leaving the microspheres, which permanently stimulate a fibrous response adding additional volume to the fill. Some redness and irritation is normal immediately after injection but resolves on its own.

The manufacturer recommends first injecting a temporary filler(HA) to the proposed area before committing to a permanent filler. To insure that the Artefill is not overdone, it is usually better if planned over several sessions. The filler is permanent and the only method of removal would be a very difficult surgical excision. The typical office preparation with a swipe of alcohol is not adequate for a permanent filler. A true surgical prep with Chlorhexadine/alcohol should be used on the skin. Artefill is not approved, and should not be used in either the lips or eyelids.

SILIKON 1000

This is an ultra pure clear silicone fluid approved by the FDA for use in eyes. Under the FDA "off label'" guideline, a practicing physician can use an approved substance in an alternative location as long as this is thoroughly explained to the patient.

Silicone injections developed a bad reputation in the past when some practitioners injected impure forms of silicone. These injections frequently led to red and lumpy areas that had to be surgically removed.

The ultra pure form is both; a permanent filler and a stimulator of a mild and predictable fibrous reaction. After injection, the fibrous reaction can take several weeks to fully enhance the fill. The filler is totally clear and can be used in areas where the color of the other fillers would show through the skin. Although it should never be used in the lips proper, many plastic surgeons are getting great results treating the rhagades[G] (smoker's lines) that radiate from the lips.

HA Filler

Physician fee[1] - $529 (see table for other fillers)

Goal of the procedure
To fill or reduce depressions from trauma or disease, such as acne.
To soften and make less visible the lines that are a part of the aging process; the

nasolabial lines, marionette lines, oral commissures, or tear trough.
To enhance the structure of the face; chin, cheeks, angle of jaw, or lips.

Alternatives

In some cases the filler is done as a temporary improvement until a facelift or mini-lift can be performed. The specific filler needs to be matched to the goal and to the area. (A reason to consider a Plastic Surgeon or Dermatologist with a full selection of choices and experience.)

Who is a good candidate?

Healthy people without allergies to the product and with realistic goals.
Blood thinners and anticoagulants will increase the risk of bruising.

Who should avoid?

Patients with a history of severe allergies.
Some fillers are not appropriate for some areas.
Patients with serious medical conditions or under treatment for cancer with chemotherapy agents.
Antimetabolite therapy such as treatment for rheumatoid arthritis.

Operator skill level (1-10) – 2 - 5

Discomfort (1-10) – 2,3

Anesthesia – Local, topical, ice or even none.

Length of procedure – 5-30 minutes depending on location and filler.

Recovery time – A few minutes of redness treated with ice. Some of the longer lasting fillers will require weeks to see final results.

Return to work - Immediately

Potential complications

Inconveniences (Level 1) – Bruising, itching, redness, pain, swelling, under or over correction.

Difficulties (Level 2) – Migration of material, tenderness, discoloration, lumps or bumps, infection at the site, rash.

Problems (Level 3) – Skin loss from compromised circulation, blindness

VERY IMPORTANT - Any loss of vision after the use of facial fillers needs IMMEDIATE transfer to an ophthalmologist or eye center.

Description of typical procedure

A topical anesthesia (dental blocks for lips) is applied to the areas to be injected and allowed 20 minutes to be effective. After a surgical prep of the area, any of several injection techniques (serial dots, threading) are used to place the filler. Massage is frequently done to the area to ensure an even distribution of the filler which is followed by ice compresses. A few minutes of icing and you can return to work.

Recovery instructions

Aggressive physical activities, alcohol and sun exposure should be avoided for one day

SPIDER VEIN Therapy (sclerotherapy)

Patients with true varicose veins, pain, and nests of large blue veins on the legs should be seen by a specialist in vascular problems. Newer methods utilizing lasers can remove them safely, with minimal scarring, and minimal risk to the deeper structures of the legs.

People with areas of small, unsightly clusters of tiny veins, commonly referred to as "spiders" or "broken veins", can be treated with micro-injections or sclerotherapy.

The solutions and techniques vary but the goal is the same. Microinjections into the vein with a sclerotherapy solution irritates the vein lining, causes swelling of the lining, which blocks the blood flow. Initially, the "spiders" look darker and more visible but that resolves within a month as the body absorbs the veins. Some solutions require a skin test for possible allergies. The type of solution, the qualification of the person doing the injection, the potential complications, and the follow-up should all be discussed prior to the procedure. Injections around the ankles are especially vulnerable to permanent brown staining (called hemosiderin) of the skin. Injections over the shin bone are the most vulnerable to skin break down and a possible permanent scar.

SCLEROTHERAPY

Physician fee[1] - $334[1]

Goal of the procedure
To reduce or eliminate unsightly spider or broken veins of the legs.
There is no actual "cure", and the goal is keeping them under control with touch-ups every few years.

Alternatives
Laser treatments, especially if you have naturally pale skin and no tan.

Who is a good candidate?
Healthy people without allergies and with realistic goals.

Who should avoid?
Patients with a history of allergies, or high dose hormonal therapy
Patients with a history of venous problems or clots.
Patients on blood thinners and anticoagulants will have decreased effectiveness of the treatment and increased risk of bruising.

Operator skill level (1-10) – 3,4

Discomfort (1-10) – 2,3

Anesthesia - None

Length of procedure – 10-20 minutes

Recovery time – The spiders typically will get darker when the blood flow stops in the tiny vessels and then resolve over the following month.
Return to work - Immediately

Potential complications
Inconveniences (Level 1) – The post treatment bandage, commonly cotton balls

and a wrap or compression stockings.

Itching, burning, redness, or swelling

Difficulties (Level 2) – Rapid recurrence, areas of discoloration (hemosiderin deposits).

Problems (Level 3) – Skin loss with a permanent scar.

Migration of the sclerosing solution into the deep venous system of the leg can cause permanent leg swelling and disability.

Description of typical procedure

Some of the solutions will cause nausea if too large a volume is used. Generally, one session is limited to about 3 cc of solution. The spiders are injected with a micro needle under magnification. Some operators prefer to foam the solution in order for the bubbles to help block the blood flow. After injection, cotton balls are taped over the treated areas and stockings or wraps applied.

Recovery instructions

On the day of the injections, you should avoid vigorous exercise, aspirins, other blood thinners, and alcohol.

The day following treatment, the wraps or stockings should be removed, the cotton balls taken off, and the wrap or stocking replaced for 2-3 more days.

Chapter Eight
The Face

"A beautiful face is a mute recommendation."
--Publillus Syrus

Your face communicates who you are to the world, sometimes accurately and sometimes not. Both the physical structure of the face and your facial expressions are broadcasting information to anyone who's tuned in. In renaissance Italy some of the first recorded Plastic Surgery procedures were to improve the physical structure of the face by rebuilding the nose. This was so important that influential patients underwent painful (anesthesia wasn't invented until 1846), prolonged (sometimes months), and dangerous or life-threatening (antisepsis wasn't invented until 1856) surgery to regain their status in society.

The Chinese *Siang Mien* masters isolated different types of faces, gave them poetic names, and assigned attributes to them:

Round faces have a keen intellect are quick witted and readily adapt to any situation. (Mao-Tse-Tung)

Diamond faces are good fighters both mentally and physically. (Madonna)

Rectangular faces are prone to introspection and have tremendous self-control. (Jennifer Aniston)

Square faces are generous and incorruptible (Churchill)

Triangular faces belong to the world's great seducers; they make up their minds quickly and don't change them. (Elizabeth Taylor)

After surveying a large group of my patients about the implications of facial characteristics and what those characteristics convey, we came up with the following list:

Sagging Brows – Stern, serious, angry

Heavy upper lids – Depressed, tired, sad

Puffy lower lids – Tired, old, drinker

Pointy Nose – Miserly, critical, superior, stingy, stern

Bulbous nose – Jovial, relaxed, drinker

Hump on Nose – Leader, rough and tumble, fighter, aggressive

Thin Lips – Gossip, angry, mad, haughty

Full Lips – Flirt, sensual, sexual

Pointy Chin – Sneaky, evil

Big boxy chin – Strong, opinionated, joker

Weak chin – Directs attention to the nose and makes it appear too large.

Short forehead – Low intelligence, gangster, impulsive

High forehead – Intelligent, curious

Downward sloping eyes – lower intelligence

Up sloping eyes – exotic, sensual

Jowls, deep facial folds, neck wrinkles – aging

Imagine the frustration if your face is communicating false messages or a message you don't want to deliver:

The young lady with puffy lower lids (probably inherited) who gets passed over for a promotion because she looks tired and stressed all the time.

The middle aged man who gets turned down for a job because his interviewer thought his round nose meant he was a drinker that didn't take life seriously.

I once did a consultation with a locally famous female trial lawyer. She was interested in reversing or reducing her signs of facial aging. As part of the consultation we discussed her brows. Her low and overhanging brows gave her a constant stern and serious look. (As you'll see later, the fix is an easy surgery with only a short time off of work.) She considered a brow lift for a while, and decided she would like the look, but that it could interfere with her career. She was concerned that her "stern and serious" look helped to get the juries attention and contributed to her success in the courtroom.

Many of these facial features can be changed or modified by Plastic Surgery, although some would be difficult. The trick is to know what your face is communicating and if that's what you want it to be communicating.

"Jeepers, creepers where'd y'a get them peepers?
Jeepers, creepers where'd y'a get those eyes?"
Lyric by Louis Armstrong

Eyelids (Blepharoplasty)

The eyes are usually considered to be the most important facial feature. When meeting someone for the first time you automatically look at is his or her eyes. By looking at someone's eyes, it opens a different level of communication with the person. Think of how annoying it is when you try to speak with someone whose eyes keep wandering. Without the eye contact, communication is so hindered that you might as well use texting (exactly what's happening). Maybe with eye contact, you really are seeing the soul, as so many poets have said. Not only are you seeing the person, you're judging them. No other part of the anatomy coveys so much information without even moving. Eyelids that are wrinkled, saggy, puffy and droopy send the message that the owner is tired, overworked, unhappy, stressed, in an unhappy relationship and/or not sleeping well.

Eyelid surgery is done less to make you look younger but more to erase the stigma of tiredness and stress. Obviously, if you're being considered for a management position, those two attributes aren't going to help your case. There can be a strong genetic component to premature changes in the eyelids. Frequently patients blame the saggy and tired eyelid changes on their parents. It's easy to appreciate why, when I can already see the same changes beginning in their five-year old daughter. The two most common age-related eyelid problems are excess and "droopy" upper eyelid skin and puffiness of the lower lid (bags). The "droopy" problem with the upper eyelid is primarily excess skin and muscle. Many people with heavy upper lids use their forehead muscles to lift the brow to take some of the pressure off of the upper lid. Unfortunately, the "frontalis" muscle isn't strong enough to do this all day long and headaches (sometimes severe) can result. My two most frequent post-operative comments after working on the upper lids are; "I can't believe that my headache is gone" and "I forgot how bright the world is".

When planning upper eyelid surgery, a consideration of the eyebrow position is essential to your surgical plan. If you're unhappy with the serious, stern look of lowered eyebrows, you probably have loose skin of their upper lids. A dangerous situation can develop if excess upper eyelid skin is removed without addressing the brow. At a later date, there may not be enough upper eyelid skin remaining to properly lift the brows and still be able to close your eyes. Conversely, it isn't unusual to do a procedure to lift the brows and discover that the lift corrected the excess upper eyelid skin.

A weak membrane holding back the fat of the lower eyelid is usually the cause of the bags and puffiness of the lower lid. As the face ages, the fat of the cheeks normally descend and the puffy lower eyelids becomes even more visible. In the past, it was common to remove fat from the lower lid to get a desirable contour. With further aging, however, this led to a "hollow" unattractive look. A newer approach to the lower lid called an "arcus marginalis release" solves that problem by retaining the fat but allowing it to blend with the cheek fat. If you're contemplating lower eyelid surgery, ask about the technique planned and do a little research. Many Plastic Surgeons consider the "arcus marginalis release" to be a significant advance.

The upper lids have a disc of cartilage for internal support that enables a more aggressive tightening of the skin. The lower lids don't have this cartilage and the expectations for tightening need to be reduced to about a 70-80% improvement. Eyelids that become increasingly "droopy" as the day progresses could have a problem with the tiny muscles that control eyelid position. They can weaken or become detached with age. Some Plastic Surgeons see enough of these cases to maintain the skill to fix this, but most don't. Ask how often your surgeon does these cases and consider asking for a referral to an Oculoplastic or Ophthalmic Plastic Surgeon.

When your mother had her eyelid surgery years ago, insurance probably paid for her upper lids. Now, insurance companies are demanding exams and objective proof that there is serious interference with vision before they even consider paying. It's still possible to get the surgery covered but at a minimum, your eye doctor will need to do a test called "visual field mapping". If you have a genuine visual problem, don't give up just because they make it more difficult.

A discussion of the "tear trough" is appropriate in your surgical plan. This is a groove extending from the corner of the eye between the nose and the cheek. If you have a unsightly deep groove, this can be treated at the time of your eyelid surgery with either transferred fat or fillers. When doing the "arcus release" it's quite easy to move some of the lower eyelid fat into the trough.

If you have a tendency to dry eyes and carry a lubricant with you, this needs to be discussed with your doctor. Everyone having eyelid surgery has some minor issues with dryness for about three months after their surgery, but, combined with a pre-existing condition, it could become serious. Medications are available to increase your tear flow, but they would need to have been started weeks prior to the surgery.

Surgery can also be used to change the lateral insertion of the eye ligaments with a dramatic change in the shape and angle of the eye. The results are so radical they should be carefully studied on a computer imaging system before making that decision. Two really bad examples of this surgery can be found among the celebrities; one a famous singer and the other an actor.

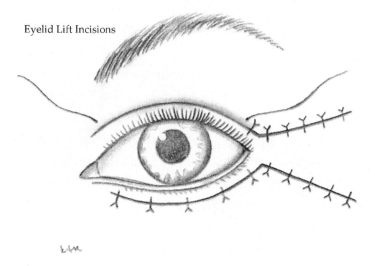

Eyelid Lift Incisions

Blepharoplasty (upper and lower)

Physician Fee[1] - $2,741 either upper or lower, discount is usual when combined.

Goal of the procedure

The goal is to create a more rested and energetic look, remove puffiness, sagging, and loose skin from the upper lids (brow would go first if needed)

Tighten and remove puffiness of the lower lids

Alternatives

There is a mechanical device that attaches to glasses to help support the upper lid. Not very successful.

Skin tightening and wrinkle improvement with lasers

Who is a good candidate?

People in good health with no significant eye disease or who are given clearance by their eye doctors.

Patients with realistic expectations and an appreciation for the limitations of the surgery.

Who should avoid?

Patients with thyroid related eye problems, severe dry eyes, glaucoma, detached retina, or other serious eye disease.

A blepharoplasty will not correct crow's feet, dark circles under the eyes (can be ethnic origin), or fine wrinkles

Operator skill level (1-10) – 4 (upper), 7(lower)

Discomfort (1-10) - 3

Anesthesia – Local with sedation or general.

Length of procedure – 45 minutes to 1 hour for uppers, same for lowers

Recovery Time – After 4 days, the sutures will be removed. Bruises will still remain 10-14 days.

Return to work – Depending on exposure to the public and makeup skills about 5 to 10 days.

Potential complications

Inconveniences (Level 1) – Swelling, burning, blurred vision, and dryness. It isn't unusual that the upper lid doesn't close completely for the first day. Use caution when first using shampoo. You may want to have baby shampoo for the first few times.

Difficulties (Level 2) – Serious bruising, bleeding, separation of the incisions, persistent blurred vision, milia^G (late formation of white heads on or near incision line)

Problems (Level 3) – Severe Dry eyes, painful irritation or scratches of the cornea, ectropion^G (separation of the lower lid from the globe), blindness, damage to the underlying muscles of the eye^{PSE} and persistent double vision^{PSE} (requires ophthalmology consult)

Description of typical procedure

You are brought to the operating room with an IV in place. The procedure is done with local and sedation or general anesthesia. The eyelids are carefully marked if not already done in the holding area. After anesthesia, two curved incisions are made in the upper lid corresponding to the amount of skin/ muscle to be removed. The upper lid is tested for excess fat, which may also be removed. Closure of the upper lids is done with very fine sutures.

The lower lids can be approached by incisions either inside the lower lid or very close to the lower lashes. Most often, the skin and muscle of the lower lids are lifted as a unit exposing the membrane holding the fat and the fat compartments themselves. After a release of the membrane (arcus marginalis release) the fat is teased across the lower bony border of the orbit and fixed in position with absorbable sutures. The lower lid skin is carefully measured and the excess skin/muscle trimmed. Wounds are closed with fine sutures and ice compresses are immediately applied.

Recovery instructions

Ice and elevation are essential for the first few days. It's much easier to prevent swelling than to get rid of it once it develops. The Internet will tell you bags of frozen peas are the ideal cold compress. You decide. You must keep your head elevated for the first few days. That could be by choosing to sleep either in a lazy boy type chair or in bed with extra pillows. Ice compresses should be applied on 15 minutes and off 15 minutes the first day while you're awake. You will have blurry vision from the ointment used by anesthesia to protect your eyes. It will clear by the second day. Move around enough to protect yourself from clots in your legs but rest. Do not do any serious physical activity, bending or heavy lifting. Bruises can get worse over the first few days. That's normal. Have on hand some artificial tears in case you need them. Do not attempt to use any makeup on the area until the sutures have been out for one day. Even then, use caution; makeup removal can be too rough for the incisions. Be very careful with contact lenses, especially hard, and how much eyelid manipulation is required to put them in and take them out.

Eyebrows

Both the Mona Lisa and the cartoon characters Wallace and Gromit have no eyebrows and still manage to communicate emotions. For the rest of us, eyebrows are not as expressive as the eyes but are still important. Raised eyebrows signify surprise, lowered eyebrows concern and seriousness. Raising one eyebrow is suspicion. About 20% of the population develop dropped eyebrows as they age. They come into the office saying, "Why are people always asking me why I'm so serious or if I'm upset?" I suffer this same condition of serious eyebrows. Once on a deep sea fishing trip, I caught a 220-pound tuna. The captain was very concerned and asked me, "Why aren't you happy? You just caught a great fish." I was going to tell him, "I really am happy, but my eyebrows are in the wrong place," but thought the better of it and let it go.

The original correction for eyebrow position was a cut from ear to ear over the top of the scalp and removal of a strip of scalp. This lift was only marginally effective while hair loss and permanent numbness was virtually guaranteed. That procedure belongs in a museum, don't do let anyone do it. It is possible to make a modest elevation of the brow by removing a small strip of skin just above the brow but the indications for that procedure are rare and the scar is permanent.

Endoscopic surgery (using a camera and scope) is now the preferred method. Whether it is done above or below the periosteum (outer covering of the bone) is still debated but surgeons get excellent results with either technique. One bonus of the endoscopic procedure is the partial removal and weakening (if desired) of the frown muscles in the space between the brows.

The procedure is frequently combined with blepharoplasty but can be done alone. The brow lift will change the tension on the upper eyelid skin and has to be done before any procedure to the upper lid.

Once the brows are lifted, some type of fixation needs to be used to hold everything in place while healing occurs. This can vary from small holes drilled in the bone, to implanted plastic anchors that slowly dissolve, to simple pins carefully drilled into the outer part of the bone. Whatever method, it needs to be flexible enough to not only lift the brow but to shape it. Many women prefer the exotic and sexy look from a little extra lift to the lateral (outer) part of the brow.

Endoscopic Brow Lift

Physician Fee[1] - $3,309[1]

Goal of the procedure
Elevation and reshaping the eyebrows to a more attractive and less angry/ serious expression. Correction of any asymmetry between brows. Secondarily, the shape of the brow can be made more exotic and the frown muscle activity reduced.

Alternatives
A tiny change in eyebrow height can be achieved with Botox laterally. There are no alternatives medially where it's most visible.

Who is a good candidate?
Patients in good health, not on blood thinners, with a good understanding of the proposed changes.

Who should avoid?
Prohibitive medical or psychological conditions.

Operator skill level (1-10) – 5,6

Discomfort (1-10) – 4,5

Anesthesia – Can be done under local with sedation but there can be a disturbing amount of noise. Frequently done with general anesthesia

Length of procedure – One hour

Recovery Time – 10 days to two weeks depending on exposure to the public and makeup skills.

Return to work – 2 days for work if you work from home, return to the workplace 10-14 days if the bruises must be resolved before you can return.

Potential complications

Inconveniences (Level 1) – Swelling, bruising, temporary numbness of the forehead

Difficulties (Level 2) – Prolonged bruising, bleeding, swelling, infection of scalp incisions, hair loss near incisions, prolonged numbness of the front of the scalp and forehead. Temporary weakness of the forehead muscles.

Problems (Level 3) – A startle or "deer in headlights" expression[PSE], permanent numbness with hair loss[PSE], asymmetry, a complete relapse of the problem. A motor nerve injury with permanent weakness of one or both sides of the forehead muscles

Description of typical procedure

In the operating room under general anesthesia, the hair is carefully separated and held with rubber bands. Five small incisions are made in the scalp inside the hairline, if possible. (one in midline, one on each side above the center of the eye, and one in each temple). These incisions are carried down to the bone and the periosteum is lifted. An endoscope is placed beneath the elevated scalp/forehead to carefully observe the nerves and avoid injury. The periosteum is released from the orbital rim and the forehead allowing the brow to become much more mobile. The brows than can be elevated or adjusted to the desired position and held in place with multiple small pins through the scalp and into the outer layer of bone or other fixation devices. If desired, small amounts of the frown muscles can be removed through the scope permanently reducing frown activity.

Scalp incisions are usually closed with staples. Bandages and drains are seldom used.

Recovery instructions

Recovery from brow surgery is similar to eyelid surgery with no heavy lifting, physical activity or bending. Ice is less important, but still indicated if you have any swelling of the eyelids. Shampoo of the scalp is possible after two or three days but the shampoo should not contain conditioners. Some caution is required not to tangle with the staples. Bruising from the browlift can take longer to appear than the eyelids but resolves in the same time frame. The staples will stay 10 to 14 days. Pins are removed on the seventh day after listening to the jokes about receiving radio stations. Bruising will usually be resolved by 10-14 days and the final result will take six weeks.

Nasal Surgery – (Rhinoplasty^G)

"A nose, kind sir! Sure, Mother Nature,
With all her freaks, ne'er formed this feature.
If such were mine, I'd try and trade it,
And swear the gods had never made it."
--Susanna Moodie

Nasal surgery is done to improve the appearance of the nose, improve breathing, or a combination of the two. Inheriting your father's nose may be fine for a young man but a young daughter may have different ideas. Although they eventually got over it, several times I've had families get angry with young ladies after a rhinoplasty. They accused her of trying to change her heritage. When operating on noses for congenital problems it's important to realize that noses have a second growth spurt that usually occurs in the early twenties. It is not unusual for someone who has only minor breathing problems to develop a more significant breathing problem in their mid-twenties. Many young people seeking improved airways have their first consultation with a Plastic Surgeon in their early twenties.

Most surgeons and surgical professors consider the Rhinoplasty to be one of the most difficult procedures in Plastic Surgery. The anatomy is complex and very small changes in the structures make huge changes in the appearance. Surgery on the nose has also been likened to flying a helicopter. Changing one thing changes all the others. My old mentor said that even though you'll be able to do an acceptable Rhinoplasty after your training, you won't be really good at it until you've been doing them for at least five years.

Computer imagining or some visual method of communication is essential when consulting about noses. There is no universally understood language that can be used to discuss nasal concerns. Many people requesting nasal surgery complain that their nose is "too long", but that expression can have very different meanings to different people.

Nasal surgery and the surgical plan need to address a multitude of different problems:

- The angle of the nose where it connects to the lip (nasolabial angle)
- The relationship of the central support of the nose (columella) as it comes from the area just beneath the nose to the top of the lip
- The nostril openings, their size and position
- The dorsum of the nose, which is where the bump would normally be
- The width and/or deviations of the dorsum of the nose
- The root of the nose, the area where the nose starts between the brows
- The nasal tip, its shape, position and relationship to the nose
- The relationship of the chin to the nose
- Internally, the septum shape and position, the turbinates which warm the air and the internal nasal valve which senses the flow of air

There is a very powerful visual relationship between the nose and the chin. About 20% of all nasal surgeries will need a chin procedure to achieve good facial balance. See the following on **Chin.**

Surgery on the nose can be done "open" with a small cut made in the columella, (the central support of the nose) and the skin of the nose lifted and turned backwards. This technique exposes the structure of the nose itself. This small cut heals very well and concerns about the scar are unwarranted. Or, the surgery on the nose can be done "closed" with all incisions done inside the nose.

Complicated noses with a history of previous surgery or difficult problems will usually be done "open". The open technique gives better exposure and better access for evaluating the situation and making the necessary corrections. Cartilage grafts are sometimes used to improve breathing or to change the shape of the nose. They are much more easily placed and anchored through the open technique. "Closed" technique can be used for the removal of a strong dorsal bump, repair of a fracture, or a refinement of the tip in an unoperated nose. Other internal surgery that improves your breathing can be done at the same time.

Nasal Anatomy

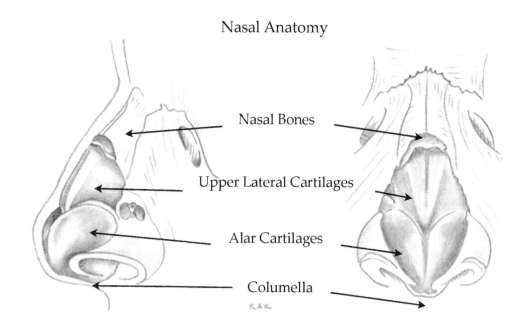

Nasal Bones

Upper Lateral Cartilages

Alar Cartilages

Columella

Nose Job (Rhinoplasty[G])

Physician Fee[1] - $4,422.00

Goal of the procedure

The surgical refinement of the nose to create an aesthetically attractive appearance, complementary facial balance, with some retained individuality.

Alternatives

Uncommonly, there are times when small amounts of fillers can accomplish the desired change.

Who is a good candidate?

Persons in good health, not on blood thinners or major medications that can identify changes that would improve their nasal esthetic. Persons with breathing problems that can be traced to a physical deformity of the nose. Persons accepting of the possibility of a second surgery to refine the procedure.

Who should avoid?

Persons who in poor health on major medications or blood thinners. Vasoconstrictors must be used inside the nose for better visibility and they may be incompatible with some cardiac conditions and treatments

Operator skill level (1-10) – 9,10

Discomfort (1-10) – 5,6

Anesthesia – Can be done with local and sedation but there is a lot of unpleasant noise. Usually General.

Length of procedure – 1.5-3 hours

Recovery Time – Bruising and swelling 10-14 days, final result 3-6 months

Return to work – One to two weeks depending on public exposure and makeup skills

Potential complications

Inconveniences (Level 1) Bruising of cheeks or eyelids, swelling, stuffiness of the nose, sinus-type headache, the nasal splint

Difficulties (Level 2) – Temporary nose bleed, packing removal (if required), recurrent deviation, supratip deformity (see note below), secondary surgery. Surgery to correct airway can take a full 3 months to notice the results.

Problems (Level 3)

Whistling after septal surgery is caused by a hole in the septum. They're not rare and can be repaired or enlarged at a later surgery. Either will stop the whistling.

Air hunger[G] can occur if certain areas of the internal nose are violated. It can be repaired but requires another procedure and grafts.

Nosebleeds, usually stop on their own within a few minutes. If not, you need to contact your doctor's office. Emergency rooms are uncomfortable with bleeding from a freshly operated nose and can cause considerable damage to the surgery.

CSF leak is a very serious problem if not recognized. There is a thin bone at the apex of the internal nose that separates the nose from the fluid surrounding the brain. Very aggressive nasal surgery or surgery on someone with a history of major facial injuries can fracture this plate. It can be recognized by a watery nasal discharge with a distinctly salty taste. Contact the doctor's office immediately.

Toxic Shock Syndrome is a rapidly progressive and potentially fatal bacterial infection associated with packing, tampons or burns. The symptoms are variable but nearly always exhibit high fever, a rapidly spreading red rash and an overall feeling of severe illness. Call your doctor **immediately** or go to an Emergency Room. If you choose the Emergency Room, let them know you had nasal surgery and have packing in place.

Description of typical (closed) procedure

Under general anesthesia in the operating room, cocaine packs are put into each side of the nose to shrink the internal membranes. Any plans to modify the nasal septum are usually completed first. This can be by making cuts to allow the septum to move, or by removing an actual portion of the septum. To access the septum the membrane covering it has to be elevated and later fixed back in place.

Incisions are made in the two lower cartilages (alar) for access to the nasal dorsum. Chisels, files and the scalpel are used to modify the nasal dorsum and sculpt the nose. After removal of the hump, the nose is probably too wide and needs to be fractured to narrow it.

Portions of the alar cartilage are removed to reshape the tip. Under some circumstances grafts may be added to rebuild the tip. Chisels or saws are used to create the nasal fracture and narrow the nose. The wound is closed with absorbable sutures and a plastic or metal splint placed on the nose to stabilize the surgery. Packing is necessary if extensive septal work is done or if there is a history of previous trauma.

Recovery instructions

After returning home, your activity is restricted, with no bending, lifting or straining. You should sleep with your head elevated by extra pillows or in a lazy boy type chair. Ice compresses can be used on the cheeks and lower eyelids. Avoid situations that can lead to sneezing like smokers or spicy cooking. You cannot blow your nose. You will have a gauze pad taped under your nose and you can change that as needed. Do not shower or get the splint wet.

Chin Procedures and Facial Implants

If you have an excessively large chin, the surgical solution will involve removal of a section of bone with stabilization of the remaining bone. The surgery has risks of healing problems, permanent loss of sensation, or alterations of the lower lip movement.

A short chin has more options. Bone grafts can be surgically inserted, the reverse of a reduction surgery, or a facial implant can be used. Long-term or permanent fillers are yet another option that can be done in the office with minimal anesthesia. Unlike the implants, fillers have the disadvantage that they can't be removed.

A safe and rapid way to augment the chin is with a chin implant. They come in a variety of shapes and sizes to accomplish nearly anything you would want. Most are made of a fully cured silicone rubber. The changes that are possible with a chin implant, just like the nose, should be reviewed on a computer imaging system. Although they can easily be removed, facial implants alter the underlying bony structure of the face and need serious consideration. It's not unusual for your family and friends to be surprised and critical of the changes immediately after surgery. I've even made patients promise to leave the implants in place for 90 days no matter what the criticism. By the end of 90 days, the chin is incorporated in your new image and the change is appreciated.

Chin Implant

Physician Fee[1] - $1,851

Goal of the procedure
Restoration of facial balance and a better facial aesthetic

Alternatives
Surgical bone grafting or fillers

Who is a good candidate?
Healthy patients with a good understanding of the changes and, ideally, a supportive family.

Who should avoid?
Patients who are unfit physically, on major medications, have cardiac conditions or require blood thinners. Patients who are unprepared for a significant alteration of their appearance.

Operator skill level (1-10) - 5

Discomfort (1-10) - 4,5

Anesthesia – General or local with sedation

Length of procedure – 30 minutes

Recovery Time – 10-14 days if bruising occurs, several months if numbness is present in the lower lip.

Return to work – 3-4 days without bruising

Potential complications
Inconveniences (Level 1) - Bruising, swelling, discomfort
Difficulties (Level 2) – Temporary numbness or weakness of the lower lip, difficulty with puckering the lips.
Problems (Level 3) – Permanent sensory nerve injury with numbness of all or part of the lower lip[PSE], permanent motor nerve injury with movement asymmetry of the lower lip[PSE], infection of the implant (requires surgical removal but can be replaced

after 3 months), the implant can shift out of position or extend over the edge of the mandible creating a visible defect

Description of typical procedure

In the operating room under general anesthesia, a three quarter inch incision is made in the upper neck following the natural groove under the chin. The incision is carried down to the front outer covering of the mandible (chin bone). The periosteum is elevated taking care to stay on the surface of the mandible and avoiding the sensory nerves. The pocket is irrigated with antibiotic solution; sizers are tried in the pocket to determine the ideal size and the permanent implant placed. Incisions are closed and tape is usually applied to stabilize the implant.

The elevated periosteum will tighten within a few days stabilizing the implant and giving the implant the feel of natural bone.

Recovery instructions

Ice compresses and an extra pillow are advisable. Heavy lifting or bending can contribute to excess bruising and should be avoided. If tape is used it needs to remain in place for one week.

Other Facial Implants

Malar Implant – put in through the lower eyelid or the mouth to augment the cheeks and give fullness to the cheekbones. In spite of going through the mouth, infections are uncommon.

Submalar Implant – Put in through the mouth, this implant can fill out the hollow that develops with aging in the area just below the cheek bones.

Orbital Rim Implant – Put in through the eyelid or mouth, this implant can help correct a "bug eyed" look when it's caused by a deficient bony structure of the orbital rim.

Mandibular Angle Implant – Put in through the mouth, this implant can augment the angle of the mandible (just beneath the earlobe) for a more masculine look to the jaw.

Nasal Implants – Can be used to strengthen the nasal dorsum or support the nasal tip. Put in through the nose, they can be problematic and extrude when used in races with thin delicate skin.

Ears

There are a number of different types of congenital ear deformities. Some are rare and difficult to fix. They should be sent to one of the handful of experts in the country who regularly works with them. The most common ear problem is children born with protruding ears. A missing fold and an excess of the scooped out portion of the ear (concha) are the most common causes. Removal of the excess concha and re-creation of the missing fold will solve most problems.

Simple protruding ears are best done at age six. At that age, the ears have had enough time to grow to be easier to work on, and its just before children get a harsh nickname that could stay with them forever. There is no maximum age and I regularly see adults who have been concealing their protruding ears with their hairdo for decades. My oldest patient was in his early sixties. He told me that he endured the nicknames throughout his school and from his children but now his grandchildren were making fun of his ears. His wife told him; "enough is enough, just go have them fixed'.

There are some promising research projects underway using small plastic night splints to reshape the ears and avoid the need for surgery. Not yet available, they show a lot of potential as a treatment option for protruding ears.

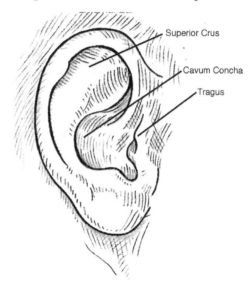

Ear Pinning (Otoplasty)

Physician Fee[1] - $3,148

Goal of the procedure

Restoration of normal appearing ears or a correction of asymmetry.

Alternatives

None (perhaps the splints in the future)

Who is a good candidate?

Children or adults in good health who will be able to wear the bandages and care for the postoperative ears.

Who should avoid?

Smokers (adults) or patients with vascular diseases that interfere with circulation.

Operator skill level (1-10) – 5,6

Discomfort (1-10) – 3,4

Anesthesia – General for children, Local with sedation or general for adults

Length of procedure – 45 minutes each ear

Recovery Time – One week if not bothered by the bruising

Return to work (school) – One to two weeks depending on tolerance of bruising. No gym or strenuous physical activities for at least 3 weeks.

Potential complications

Inconveniences (Level 1) – Bruising, swelling, itching or mild discomfort. The need to wear a head bandage initially and then a headband to protect the ears

Difficulties (Level 2) – Prolonged bruising or swelling, infection, irritation of the ear canal (could be caused by blood in the canal),

Problems (Level 3) – Partial or complete recurrence of the deformity. Unnatural look, asymmetry between the two ears, "telephone ear" where the central portion of the ear is overcorrected while the earlobe and top portion of the ear still protrude[PSE], it is correctable but requires additional surgery. Abnormal scarring of the cartilage. Keloids or healing problems.

Description of typical procedure (child)

Patient is taken to the OR and given general anesthesia. Local anesthesia is also used to reduce bleeding and make the surgery easier. The incision is made inconspicuously behind the ear with only a small incision on the front. Through the front incision, scratches are made on the surface of the cartilage to weaken it and make the new fold easier to create. From behind, the new enhanced crease is reinforced with sutures. If any excess conchal[G] cartilage needs to be removed, its marked, excised and the defect sutured closed. After a careful comparison of both ears, the wounds are closed and bandages applied. The first bandage will likely be a full head bandage.

Recovery instructions

Bandages must remain in place for the first few days. Activities are restricted, especially those that could result in the accidental removal of the bandages. Tylenol is usually the only medication needed for discomfort. After 5 days the bandage is removed in the office and replaced with a soft headband worn over top of the ears, not above them. The headband should be continued for several weeks depending on the reliability and aggression of the child.

Neck Lift

The neck lift is a frequently requested procedure that I infrequently do. The neck is just one of the visible signs of aging, even though it may be the most visible. Other signs include deepening of the nasolabial fold[G], formation of the marionette lines[G], jowls, and hollowness of the cheeks. Doing a neck lift as an isolated procedure, can improve the neck at the expense of accentuating the jowls and exaggerating the other effects of aging. In consultation, once these things are pointed out to the patient, most will opt for a more comprehensive procedure that addresses all the problem areas.

Rarely, I do sometimes see people who have excess fat and/or skin of the neck without the other signs of advancing age. In the past, surgeons liberally used liposuction in the neck to remove fatty deposits and reshape it. The problem was that it didn't always work. Research found that in a significant percentage of people the excess neck fat can be underneath the outer sheet of muscle where liposuction can't reach it. The solution is to make a small cut under the chin, look to see where the fat is located, and manually remove it if under the muscle.

Neck-bands generate some disagreement among Plastic Surgeons. Some recommend cutting them, others sew them together; still others combine cutting and sewing. All of these techniques work in skilled hands but you might want to ask your surgeon what his plan is. My old mentor used to say; "If there's more than three ways to do something, either they all work or none of them do."

Not everyone can have a long, sculpted neck. There is a bone in the neck that sets the neck angle and anchors some of the muscles of the tongue and neck. The position of that bone (hyoid) determines the neck angle and cannot be changed.

Neck Lift

Physician Fee[1] – Not Available as an isolated procedure.

Goal of the procedure
Restore the contour of the neck, tightening of the skin, reduction of excess fat and elimination of the neckbands.

Alternatives
Consider a facelift or mini facelift for more effective improvement, longer

duration and overall aesthetic. Fraxel lasers can have a modest effect but the neck is a dangerous area for resurfacing either by laser or chemical peel.

Who is a good candidate?

Healthy people, non-smokers, not on blood thinners, with an understanding of the aging process and the desire to improve the neck.

Who should avoid?

Smokers, patients with serious medical conditions, patients with unrealistic expectations

Operator skill level (1-10) – 5,6

Discomfort (1-10) - 5

Anesthesia – Local with sedation or general

Length of procedure – 1 – 1 ½ hours

Recovery Time – 10 – 14 days although some lumpiness and hardness will persist up to 3 months.

Return to work - 10 – 14 days, but shorter with minimal exposure to the public and good makeup skills

Potential complications

Inconveniences (Level 1) Bruising, stiffness, minor swelling, presence of a drain, sometimes a cervical collar.

Difficulties (Level 2) Hematoma[G] (collection of blood in the neck), prolonged hardness or stiffness, color changes of the skin

Problems (Level 3) Skin loss with resultant scarring (most commonly behind the ears in smokers), motor nerve injury[PSE] (permanent or temporary) causing a distortion of the mouth with animated speech, hoarse voice from a different nerve injury[PSE], Breathing difficulty can be caused by excess swelling or bleeding under the skin (a life threatening emergency, don't hesitate to get treatment)

Description of typical procedure

You would be taken to the OR and under anesthesia or sedation; local is placed in the neck to reduce bleeding. The first incision is usually just beneath the chin to expose the muscle bands and/or fat of the submental area. Neckbands are sutured together or cut and the excess fat removed. Incisions are made behind each ear and the skin elevated to the midline. Carefully balancing the sides, the excess skin is trimmed, a drain or two is put in place and the wounds are closed. Some surgeons prefer a bandage or a cervical collar to support the skin during the initial phases of healing.

Recovery instructions

Elevation of the head neck area for the first few days will help to minimize swelling. Ice compresses should be used in moderation. The skin is fragile and excess ice can damage it. Avoid lifting, bending or straining.

There are some "thread" variations that are less invasive (and less effective). They utilize threads crisscrossing the neck to improve the angle and elevate the skin. These procedures don't allow removal of any excess skin and probably have the most application for young people. Thread lifts are designed as an office procedure to keep down the costs and inconvenience. Using threads for a facelift has a sketchy past. Most of those techniques are no longer done because of a rapid recurrence of the problem or because they can leave palpable nodules beneath the skin. If your doctor is recommending thread-type facelift, be cautious and do your homework.

The neck lift would be considered a "mini-lift" because it addresses one area only. Other "mini-lifts" can be done for the midface, the jawline, or the forehead (discussed).

Face Lift (Rhytidectomy[G])

The facelift is one of the hallmark operations of Plastic Surgery and one that attracts the most attention. The facelift procedure really came into its own when creative surgeons incorporated lessons learned from treating war wounds into the cosmetic side of Plastic Surgery. Early attempts at facelifting removed small patches of skin to tighten and "lift" the face. Some success was achieved, as evidenced by early photographs. The problem was the durability. Skin-only lifts quickly stretch the skin and relapse. Pulling harder on the skin only increases the scarring and the risk of poor healing. Words of caution, some of the "lunch-time lifts" are a big step backwards with a skin-only lift.

One of the first female Plastic Surgeons, Suzanne Noel, practiced in France between the two World Wars and left us excellent records. She used small clips similar to clothespins to pinch the areas of excess facial skin and preview the improvement. Once she and her patients were satisfied, she surgically removed the pinched skin and repaired the wounds. Her results were very good but her recurrence must have been very rapid.

A major improvement occurred when the SMAS[G] (Superficial Muscular Aponeurotic System) was identified and incorporated into the facelift. This layer beneath the skin and above the muscles has enough strength to be lifted separate from the skin and is fibrous enough to resist stretch better than the skin. With only one exception, all modern facelifts incorporate some version of the SMAS lift.

SMAS Facelift

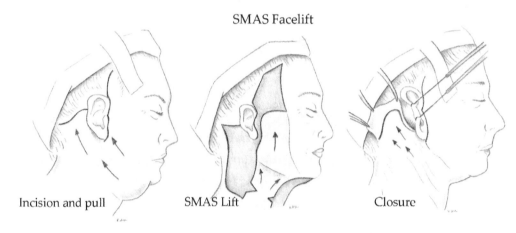

Incision and pull   SMAS Lift   Closure

The exception is the Deep Plane Facelift, which lifts the face, muscles and structures off of the facial skeleton and repositions them. The surgery is complicated, time consuming, and challenging. The results can be dramatic. It has never achieved wide-spread acceptance because of the extensive swelling and prolonged recovery period (sometimes as much as long as six months before the swelling finally resolves).

"A facelift will erase about 10 years of aging and will last about 10 years," is probably the most often heard explanation of a facelift from Plastic Surgeons. But, what does it mean? It could mean that after 10 years you would be back to the look that caused you to decide on the facelift in the first place. It could mean that many people repeat their facelift at ten years. What it doesn't mean is that at the end of ten years (similar to Cinderella) you wake up and everything is gone. My personal favorite explanation; If you had an identical twin and you underwent a facelift and they didn't. At the conclusion of the facelift you would look ten years younger than your twin. As you both continue to age, you will continue to look ten years younger.

Smokers are not good candidates for a facelift. Smokers have ten times the risk of a serious complication (problem) compared to non-smokers. When smokers come to me for a facelift, I require a minimum of three weeks smoke free before surgery. One of two days before the surgery, I test their urine for smoking byproducts and if positive, I cancel their case. If they live with another smoker, they need to work out a system in advance that the patient is never confined with a smoker. Watch out for smoke in the car. Facial skin, after it has been elevated in a facelift, is fragile. It can be damaged by pressure (swelling or hematoma[G]) or the effects of smoking. Smoking produces chemicals in your blood that constrict the tiny blood vessels keeping the skin healthy. The final outcome of smoking after a facelift can be a loss of skin requiring multiple additional surgeries and a prolonged recovery time.

SMAS Facelift

Physician Fee - $6,426

Goal of the procedure
Facial rejuvenation by lifting and tightening the facial skin (and deeper structures), softening of the nasolabial lines and marionette lines, more fullness to the midface and cheeks, smoother and less wrinkled neck. A more rested and relaxed appearance.

Alternatives
Some improvement can be obtained with laser resurfacing.

Who is a good candidate?

Healthy patients, non-smokers, free of serious cardiac or significant illness. Able to appreciate the proposed surgery

Who should avoid?

Perfectionists, smokers, severe chronic illness sufferers, people with unrealistic expectations about the surgery and the anticipated social ramifications of the surgery. Patients on blood thinners or who cannot tolerate the anesthetic agents.

Operator skill level (1-10) - 5–9 (not hard to do the procedure, hard to do well)

Discomfort (1-10) – 3-5

Anesthesia – Local with sedation or General
Length of procedure – 3-4 hours

Recovery Time – 10-14 days

Return to work – 10-14 days depending on public exposure and makeup skills

Potential complications
Inconveniences (Level 1)

Bruising, swelling, numbness, drains, pressure or tightness.

Difficulties (Level 2)

Excessive bleeding or malfunctioning drain, persistent numbness, swelling or bruising. temporary hair loss, poor healing behind the ears, irregularity of the skin, discoloration of the skin.

Problems (Level 3)

Unnatural look with poor animation or asymmetry of the face

Loss of earlobe from poor technique[PSE]

Loss of sideburn or temple hair[PSE]

Excessive forehead[PSE]

Distortion of the little bump in front of the ear (Tragus[G])[PSE]

Joker lines – caused by incorrect vectors when setting the skin in a facelift. They are lines or folds from the corner of the mouth obliquely extending toward middle or top of the ear.[PSE]

Permanent hair loss[PSE]

Permanent numbness of the earlobe (a nerve injury)

Permanent muscle weakness or paralysis. Forehead, and corner of the mouth are the most common.

Skin loss with scarring (neck and behind the ear are most common) (most common in smokers but can occur in non-smokers.

Description of typical procedure

You will be taken to the OR and after rearranging the beds you will either have general anesthesia or sedation with local. Regardless, local has to be used to minimize bleeding. If eyelid or brow surgery is included, that would be done first. I like to begin with the neck. Incisions are made in the hair of the temple taking care to keep the incisions angled the same as the hairs for minimal damage. The incision is carried down in front of the ear, curves below the earlobe and traces the back of the ear into the hair. A second incision is made in the submental area just beneath the chin. Any planned liposuction or fat removal of the neck is done. The skin of the neck is carefully elevated from the center out and from behind the ears toward the midline. Any adjustments needed to the neckbands can be done by cutting or banding them together. Attention is then directed to raising the facial skin. Experience and caution allows the surgeon to stay in exactly the right level. The skin is generally elevated to just short of the NL line and stops when the orbital muscles of the eye become visible.

Three nerves have to be avoided at this level, one supplies movement to half of the forehead, another movement to the mouth corner and the third is the sensory nerve to the earlobe.

The next step is a cautious elevation of the SMAS^G . Once elevated, it can be tightened and manipulated to the ideal vector^G needed to accomplish the rejuvenation goal. Because of its fibrous nature and deeper position, more tension can be put on the SMAS than the skin would tolerate. Drains are placed beneath the skin flaps, which are lifted and rotated to the ideal position and sutured in place without tension. Drains only stay 24 hours, and although many surgeons use bandages, I never do.

Closure in the hair-bearing areas must respect the angles of the hairs or baldness can result. Closure near the earlobe must be free of tension or the earlobe will be distorted and blend into the cheek and create an "operated look". Closure behind the ear is delicate, this is the most fragile skin and should have no tension in the final layer. This is also the most likely site for unsatisfactory scarring.

You are transferred to recovery keeping your head elevated and using intermittent ice compresses. Discharge home when recovery criteria are met.

Recovery instructions

You need to rest with your head in an elevated position either with extra pillows or in a last boy type chair. Watch the drains carefully and empty as necessary. Ice compresses can be used for swelling but not as aggressively as the eyelids. Continue the compression stockings for the first full day to help protect against blood clots. Bleeding is the biggest concern in the immediate postoperative period. Sudden rapid swelling of one side of the face accompanied by an increase in pain could be bleeding and warrants an immediate call to your surgeon's office (any hour!). Many patients choose to engage a private duty nurse or have an overnight arrangement with a surgical facility. They can help with compresses, pain meds and generally add a level of security that relieves your family of a lot of anxiety. The drains are removed the next day and sutures removed at 5, 7, and 10 days.

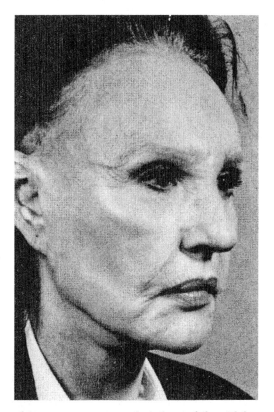

Facelift Errors; a bizarre appearance, hair loss of the sideburns and temple, exaggerated forehead height, distorted tragus, stretched earlobe, and loss of normal facial contours. (Used by permission Dr. Thomas J Baker)

MACS Lift (Minimal Access Cranial Suspension)

One of the most successful mini-lifts was developed in Belgium and is known as the MACS Lift, which stands for Minimal Access Cranial Suspension. Instead of elevating the SMAS layer like a traditional facelift, the procedure uses sutures to fold (plicate) the SMAS into pleats that heal together for long-term durability. The incision is much smaller and the overall procedure is faster. Another significant feature of this "mini-lift" is the vertical nature of the lift. A SMAS lift will have it strongest pull at an angle toward the top of the ear. The MACS lift creators say that angle is wrong and is not the direction of aging. Gravity and aging are Down so the direction of the MACS Lift is Up. This is a very good lift for younger people interested in "heading off" the signs of aging. It isn't as useful for older patients who need the removal of significant amounts of skin.

MACS Lift

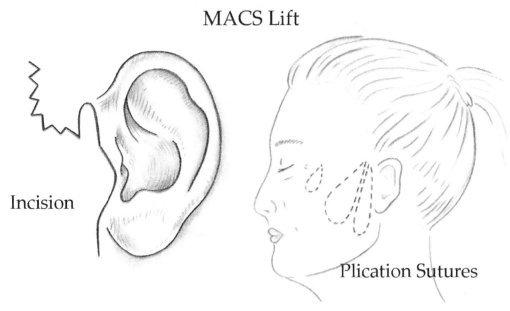

Incision

Plication Sutures

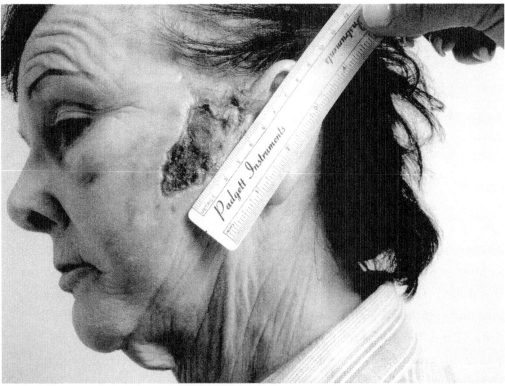

"A healthy 69 yo 5 weeks after a mini facelift. She was excellent at three weeks, this scar occurred in the fourth and fifth week after exposure to cigarette smoke by her family. She required multiple procedures."

Chapter Nine
The Breasts

Women are always complaining about men's fascination with breasts.
But what if men were absolutely indifferent to breasts?
What would women do then with these things that serve one function once or twice in a lifetime, then the rest of the time are just in the way?
--Jonathan Carroll

With Great Breasts Comes Great Responsibility
Darynda Jones, Second Grave on the Left (T-shirt)

Breast

Breast surgery is the most common Plastic Surgery procedure according to the 2011 ASPS survey data with over 500,000 cases performed annually. Augmentation mammoplasty accounts for over 300,000 of these procedures. Breast surgery, paradoxically, has both some of the highest satisfaction numbers, over 87% and severe dissatisfaction, leading to the highest number of successful malpractice suits. Clearly, this is an area of Plastic Surgery where better decisions can make a huge difference.

The possible cosmetic breast procedures include:

- Enlargement (augmentation mammoplasty[G])
- Reducing the size for females (reduction mammoplasty[G])
- Reducing the size for males (gynecomastia[G] correction)
- Lifting the breasts (mastopexy[G])
- Lesser procedures; correction of inverted nipples, nipple reduction, or liposuction of the axillary tail of the breast

Breast augmentation illustrates two concepts we talked about earlier:

- It's easy to do the surgery, but difficult to do the surgery well.
- The practices with the highest volume have the least problems.

To those, I would add a third:

- If breast augmentation is only a minor part of a practice and the current procedure is producing an "acceptable" result, there is little incentive to learn the newer techniques and products.

How else can you explain American docs who continue to tell their patients; "Saline implants are the safest and most natural implants."? This isn't true, and hasn't been true for over a decade.

Augmentation Mammoplasty

In November 2006, The FDA released the silicone implant for surgical use after a 14-year ban. After all of that time, there was never any conclusive evidence linking the implants to any disease. In sympathy, the FDA equivalent organizations around the world also banned the silicone implant. Most of those organizations released the silicone implant for use in six months to a year (not 14 years). A 14-year ban meant that large numbers of new Plastic Surgeons completed their training and went into practice without ever working with the silicone implant.

The silicone implant first came on the market in the US in 1962. At that time the FDA did not have authority over medical devices. That changed, and the FDA, after they were mandated that responsibility, began requiring proof of "safety and efficacy" from medical device manufacturers. The manufacturers at the time of the ban were not forthright about providing this information and were given warnings from the FDA. About this time, a media frenzy of "alleged" implant atrocities took over all the national news and ultimately forced the FDA to the ban. Although always considered softer and more natural feeling than saline, the old silicone implant had several problems prior to the ban. They included; an unknown rate of rupture, poor quality liquid silicone filler, inflammation and scar formation if ruptured, and high levels of platinum in some of the manufacturing processes. Why the ban lasted 14 years and why the eventual approval was limited to age 22 and above, is anyone's guess.

Saline Implant

Outside the United Stated, the saline implant has limited application and is rarely used except for special circumstances. A few advantages to the saline are; that it's adjustable, it can be inserted through a small incision, and it can be inflated in place. A partial list of the disadvantages include; a failure rate of 50% within 10 years, a heavier and less natural feeling implant, and a higher tendency to ripples and wrinkles, and a virtually necessity to use it beneath the muscle (sub-pectoral).

Cohesive Gel Implant

While the United States was in the 14 year breast Dark Ages, the French reinvented the silicone implant. Chemists addressed the primary problems of the old silicone implant and solved them. The tendency to silent rupture was improved with newer materials and better manufacturing processes. Most importantly, the inflammation and scarring sometimes caused by leaking liquid silicone was solved with a purer grade of silicone and a different type of gel that doesn't leak. The silicone filler material was re-engineered with more chemical cross-links to form a thicker (more "cohesive") gel that won't spill out or leak even if the implant is injured. The superior softness and natural feel of the old silicone implants has been made even better with the new implants. Called "cohesive gel" implants for the newer type gel center, marketers called it the "gummy-bear implants" and, of course, the name stuck. Already the most successful implant in most of the world, the United States is rapidly catching up.

The 90-day Phenomenon.

Numerous psychiatrists and psychologists have undergone breast augmentation procedures over the years. A surprising majority of them agree on this phenomenon. For the first 90 days when you look in the mirror, you see yourself with artificial breasts. But, on day 91, the new breasts have been incorporated into your self image and you see yourself looking back. It seems that a cosmetic procedure which turns back time to a look you used to have (facelift) is accepted immediately into your self-image. When a change creates an entirely new you, (chin implant, breast augmentation) the 90 day rule takes affect.

The Four Decisions of Breast Augmentation

1. Type of Implant

Saline Implant

Advantages– The implant is less expensive, approved for use in patients as young as 18, uses a smaller incision for placement, and is size adjustable.

Disadvantages – The saline implant has a 50% failure rate in 10 years, a higher risk of wrinkles or ripples, it must be used under the muscle in most applications, its heavier and less natural feeling with no ability to hold a shape. (it adjusts to where it's placed.)

Cohesive gel implant (Gummy Bear)

Advantages – It is a softer, lighter, and more natural feeling implant. It can be used in any of the locations. The implant is shape-stable, and will maintain its shape in any position. It has a longer durability and resistance to injury (one company has a lifetime replacement warranty). It has less risk or wrinkles or ripples.

Disadvantages – Only approved for use at age 22 and above, slightly more expensive, and is pre-filled with no adjustability and more limited size options.

2. Incision

Axillary – There is a minimal risk of reduced nipple sensation, and a moderate risk of infection. Because of the limited incision size without the scar becoming visible, it is nearly impossible to fit even a modest sized CG implant through this incision. It does give a cosmetically good scar.

Umbilical – The only advantage to this technique is in the marketing. One series at a well-known east coast university reported a 25% incidence of implant malposition requiring additional surgery. The procedure can only be done with deflated saline implants and even then, it voids the implant warranty.

Periareolar – Placement of the implant through a cut partially around the areola. Unless the areola is large, again, it may not be possible to fit a CG implant through the incision. This approach has both an increased risk of decreased nipple sensation and an increased risk of infection. I usually recommend against this incision if there is a chance for future breast-feeding. Cosmetically the scar can be good.

Inframammary Fold – The implant is placed through a cut in the crease beneath the breast. Cosmetically this approach gives a excellent scar with the least risk of either infection or change of nipple sensation. The incision location gives good access for either subfascial or subpectoral placement without causing damage to the muscle. It is also a good incision and good access for revision work.

3. Implant Location

Subglandular – The subglandular position refers to the placement of the implant above the muscle but below the breast tissue. This position gives the maximum amount of lift to the breast with an implant alone, but has the highest risk of wrinkles or ripples showing. It is usually reserved for early ptosis in a patient with a moderate amount of natural breast volume. Ladies who are already a "C" cup and are going to "D" or "DD" do very well with this procedure.

Subpectoral – The placement of the implant partially beneath the pectoralis muscle of the chest. This placement gives the maximum protection from ripples or wrinkles at the top and middle of the breast, but the least amount of lift. The final result will sometimes have a troublesome "motion artifact" with visible movement of the breast when using the chest muscles. It can be disastrous to trainers and professional athletes who either stand in front of exercise classes or are physically active on camera. I had one professional golfer who came to me requesting that I move her implants to above the muscle. The cameraman told her he couldn't shoot her because the camera picked up the jump of her breast every time she made a swing.

Full muscle coverage is possible by incorporating other chest wall muscles but is rarely done except for breast reconstructions.

Subfascial – A procedure, not yet popular in the US, that was developed in Brazil. The implant is placed beneath the outer covering of the pectoralis muscle (called "fascia"). The position offers good resistance to ripples and wrinkles and simultaneously affords good lift to correct early sagging. Motion artifact does not occur. It can be a difficult procedure to learn. After talking to the developer of this procedure (Dr. Ruth Graf) in Brazil, I was convinced of the merits of this technique and immediately began using it when I returned home. My first few procedures took three times as long as normal with more bleeding, but by the 6th procedure, my surgical times were the same as the other two methods with no excess bleeding.

4. Size of the Implant

Size can be chosen by computer imaging, experimenting with bags of rice at home, trying on the implants in a bra, or (our method) trying sizers filled with polyethylene beads in a stretch bra with a built-in pocket. We developed these sizers because we felt that computer imaging distorts the nipple areola complex and gives a surreal look to the breasts. The bags of rice are too heavy and sit too low on the chest, and using actual implants in a bra give a false idea of projection. Using sizers with beads in a stretch bra overcomes all of these issues, and patients using this method of sizing have an exceptionally high patient satisfaction rate.

Some practices take measurements of your chest and plug these into a formula that tells you what size implant you should use (the engineers at work).

Their mathematical model permits only a small amount of flexibility and may not give you the look that you want.

South American Plastic Surgeons and some practices in the US use "sizers" in the operating room. After the surgical pocket has been created, the doctor will try different size sizers until he/she has what they believe is the "best look" for you, then put in the permanent implant. Their idea of a "best look" may not be anything near your goal. I was dumbfounded a few years ago at a conference in Brazil to hear a serious discussion between two Plastic Surgeons on whether or not the patient has the right to choose the size of their implants. I believe this is wrong on two levels:

First, I think that patient's wishes need to be discussed, respected and given primary consideration well before going to the operating room, accepting that, occasionally, patients ask for procedures that are either impossible or inappropriate. If a compromise in the surgical plan can't be reached with additional consultation time, then you should be denied.

Second, it is well established in Plastic Surgery that minimal or "no touch" technique for placement of the implant reduces the risk of complications. By touching sizers (maybe several), putting them in and out of the pocket, and then their removal and replacement with a permanent implant, there is a much higher likelihood of bacterial contamination which can lead to complications.

I frequently see unhappy patients in my office that thought they had good communication with their surgeon and an agreement on the implant size only to wake up and find that their surgeon put in a much larger implant than expected. The explanation given is usually "when I got in there, I felt this would be a better size for you." Are you kidding?

Just a couple days ago, a patient came to my office who was asked by the surgical assistant in another office (not even the doctor) what range of implant sizes she was interested in. That way, in surgery, the Doctor could choose which size was best for her. She had already put down a deposit but demanded the money back, cancelled the case and came to my office. If everyone had that courage, there would be less need for a book like this.

A tip: When you're looking at a computer or trying on some type of sizing in the doctor's office, look at your shoulders as they relate to your proposed breasts. Just as the nose / chin relationship is critical to the apparent size of the nose, the breast / shoulder relationship is important if your goal is to have a natural look. If you're going for outrageous, just ignore this. Don't get confused trying to match your breast size with your hips. Millions of women have mismatched upper and lower bodies, and whole clothing lines have grown up based on selling the tops and bottoms separately. When someone is watching you on the beach in your new bikini and trying to guess if they're real or plastic, chances are they're looking (without realizing it) at the relationship between your shoulders and your "girls".

"Vanity sizing" has come to bras. When new patients ask me what bra size she would be after her augmentation, my response is; "Where do you buy your bras?" Women have been living with "vanity sizing" for years. You all know that better quality shoes or dresses will have a smaller size written on the label. Now, the same has happened to bras, some stores are miss-sizing their bras, allegedly, to make you feel better about yourself. Consider a variation of the old adage, "If it walks like a duck, looks like a duck and sounds like a duck, it's probably a duck." If it looks like a "C" cup and feels like a "C" cup then it's probably a "C" cup even if the shop girl at Victoria's Secret swears you're a "DD". For men, if you're going to give lingerie for a present, get a return receipt.

5. Shape of the Implant

The choice of shape with saline implants is meaningless. A non shape-stable implant will fill the space it's put into and be shaped by the skin and the muscles. Shape-stable or cohesive gel implants come with different projections and shapes. The shape outside of the body is maintained after surgical placement. Implants with a superior extension or "tear drop" shape can be used to compensate for minimal chest musculature or to produce more fill in the upper pole of the breast. Implants with higher projection allows more volume for women with narrow chests.

Don't be surprised if you hear the word "footprint" when discussing the cohesive gel implants. Remember, cohesive gel implants maintain their shape inside the body as well as outside. Studies from countries that have had these implants much longer than the US find that the base diameter, or "footprint", of the implant must closely correlate with the actual breast to give the most natural appearance. An implant too wide will project into the armpit and one that's too narrow will look artificial.

When I'm having an implant discussion with a pre-operative patient I tell them that first we have to get the footprint right and then we can see what's possible. The designers of these implant have done a good job and there will be a lot of choices. With a reasonable chest width, "B" cup to "DD" cup is probably possible. If you want "Texas or Dolly size", it may not be possible with the cohesive implants because of the footprint. You might have to go to a liquid filled implant to get the supersizes.

Bilateral Augmentation Mammoplasty

Physician Fee - $3,388

Goal of the procedure

To restore or create natural appearing and feeling breasts that balance with the shoulders and sometimes add a little extra.

Alternatives

There is a vacuum device worn on the chest at night that will give a modest increase in size. It's cumbersome, expensive, slow and the results can be disappointing.

For people who still have implant safety concerns, fat injections to augment the breast are gaining in popularity. (More to follow)(Problems include the need for multiple injections and the concern that the fat grafts could interfere with future mammograms.)

Who is a good candidate?

Most patients fall into one of two categories: Young ladies who have never been satisfied with their breasts that now have enough expendable income and time to have augmentation surgery. Or, ladies who are finished having children, lost breast tissue, and now want their bodies back.

Age 18+ for saline and 22+ for cohesive gels, although there can be exceptions.

Who should avoid?

Women who are actively breast-feeding. The breasts take a full 3 months to normalize after breast-feeding.

Women with a planned weight loss of 15 or more pounds.

Patients with risk of cancer need to discuss the options with your doctor. This isn't an absolute contraindication, but a few things can be done differently. Putting the implants under the muscle will spare the natural breast any trauma and present the least problems if cancer later develops in the breast. In some very high-risk circumstances, a partial mastectomy with immediate implants can reduce the risk of cancer and an acceptable aesthetic result. (The skin and nipple are retained but the breast substance is removed and replaced with an implant.)(it is sometimes called the 95% mastectomy)

Breast Augmentation has powerful psychological implications and your surgeon needs to spend some time getting to know you and your goals. The woman who comes in wanting larger breasts to save a foundering marriage may do better with counseling or a divorce attorney, while the recently divorced woman may just get the self confidence boost she needs to begin dating again.

Operator skill level (1-10) – 6,7

Discomfort (1-10) – 2-7 depending on the implant placement and size

Anesthesia - General

Length of procedure – 1 – 1 ½ hours

Recovery Time – 3 weeks

Return to work – 3 days for desk job, 5-7 days for moderate physical requirements 2-3 weeks for police, psychiatric or emergency room nurses

Potential complications

Inconveniences (Level 1)

Discomfort, swelling, unnatural temporary elevation of the implant (with sub-pectoral), increased sensitivity of the nipple, asymmetry (one implant will always take longer to settle into position), a sensation of water moving, or occasional sharp pains

Difficulties (Level 2)

Ripples or wrinkles in the implant, prolonged elevation or asymmetry of the implants on the chest wall, hematoma or seroma, infection, loss of nipple sensitivity, difficulty accepting the new "look" (remember the 90 day rule), erection or hardness of the nipple (can last several months)

Problems (Level 3)

Capsular Contracture with elevation, hardness and discomfort of the implant. (see note below.)

Exposure of the implant[PSE] will almost certainly result in the loss of the implant

Permanent loss of nipple sensation.

Malposition of one or both implants is usually a surgical error:

Symmastia[GPSE] – when the implants merge in the middle creating one large breast with outward pointing nipples.

Bottoming Out[G] – when the implant descends on the chest below the natural inframammary fold. The nipples will turn up, called "stargazers".

Lateral Displacement – when the implants move toward the armpits and the nipples face straight ahead (headlights[G]).

Description of typical procedure

You are taken to the Operating room and after some table adjustments, anesthesia is administered, either general or sedation with local. Marks are placed to indicate the midline, the inframammary fold and the incision. For cohesive gel implants, the incision is 1.5 inches for small to moderate implants and 2 inches for large implants. Protective plastic sheets are put in place over the nipples. The incision is carried down to the lower edge of the Pectoralis muscle. The implant pocket can be developed above the fascia (subglandular), below the fascia (subfascial) or below the muscle (subpectoral). After completing the pocket and assuring there is no bleeding, the pocket is irrigated with an antibiotic mixture. Implants are then placed with "No or Minimal touch" technique. Symmetry is carefully checked and the wounds closed in multiple layers with glue on the skin surface.

Patients are generally placed in a light bandage, bra, and chest strap before being transported to the recovery area.

Recovery instructions

Bra and strap are worn 24/7 for the first few days except for brief showers. Gentle stretch exercises begin before discharge and continued for the first few weeks. There are no bandages to changes. You may shower the same day as the surgery after a brief nap. For the first week after the surgery, activity is limited to lifting 15 pounds or less. The second week, you can go above the 15 pounds but avoid anything bouncy (jogging, motorcycles, jet skis or horseback riding). The third week, you may resume all activities.

We have two different protocols for the management of discomfort. The first is non-narcotic. We give a medication that alters the pain threshold (Lyrica) in combination with a high dose of Ibuprophen (Motrin). Over 90% of our patients do well with this protocol and appreciate not having to deal with the problems of narcotics. The second protocol utilizes a traditional narcotic in moderate dosage.

Capsular Contracture is the most common serious complication of augmentation mammoplasty. It can occur weeks or years after your surgery. Different studies list the incidence at variously 3% to almost 50%. Theories on the origin of capsular contracture have ranged from leaking silicone from the implants, to the position of the implant, to the covering or texture of the implant. Increasing evidence implicates a recently identified type of slow lingering infection called a biofilm. Biofilms are known to be problematic with other indwelling medical devices such as orthopedic prosthesis, catheters, and artificial heart valves may be one of the major causes of capsular contracture. Biofilms are difficult to identify, and expensive to prove, but there are steps that can be taken to minimize their occurrence. Specific skin preps, antibiotic irrigations, and minimal handling of implants all reduce the risk. Marginally effective treatments for capsular contractures include ultrasound, vitamin E, massage and several types of asthma medications. If all of these fail to offer any improvement, the definitive treatment is surgical but requires several specific steps. If you're having surgery for a capsular contracture, you need to know the surgical plan and discuss these steps with your surgeon. If he/she doesn't agree, consider changing surgeons.

1. The implant must be removed and replaced; it cannot be reused or resterilized.

2. All traces of the capsule must be removed unless removal would constitute an unacceptable health hazard, such as a capsule stuck to the thin muscle layer between the ribs. The old recommendation of a cut in the capsule (capsulotomy) has an unacceptably high rate of recurrence.

3. Gloves must be changed or rinsed with antibiotic solution prior to touching the new implants.

4. Chlorhexadine alcohol is the preferred skin prep.

5. OpSite or plastic sheeting should be placed over the nipples prior to starting the procedure.

6. "No Touch" or minimal touch technique must be practiced.

7. The triple antibiotic rinse recommended by Dr. Adams and the Dallas group   should be used to soak the implant prior to insertion and to rinse the pocket.

8. In spite of the fact that the Dental associations and Family Practice associations do not recommend it. We recommend the same antibiotic prophylaxis that the American Heart Association does for Dental cleanings and "dirty" surgical procedures. ("dirty" surgical procedures in this case, are procedures which cause bleeding in areas which cannot be properly cleaned or disinfected ie. mouth, vagina, anus, rectum).

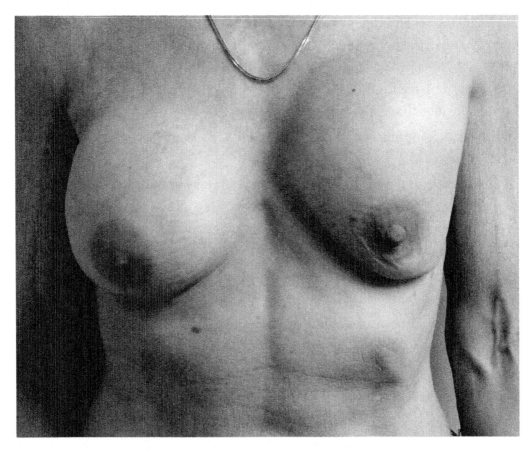

CC 61 yo with Severe breast capsular contracture.

Fat Grafting for Augmentation

Fat grafting for the breast is a controversial technique that utilizes your own fat to increase the size and volume of the breast or change the shape. It must be done over multiple sessions to achieve any significant size change. The addition of the chest vacuum pump permits more fat to be successfully grafted at each session. The apparatus consists of a fiberglass shell, which is worn over the breasts every night, and attached to a vacuum. The application of suction to the breasts opens up spaces in the breast, increases circulation, and permits larger graft survival.

Critics of the procedure claim that it is slow, cumbersome, minimally effective and expensive. But most importantly, critics claim that on mammograms, the fat grafts look very similar to early stage breast cancer.

Advocates claim that radiologists who read the mammograms can learn to spot the differences between fat grafts and cancer. They also promote the concept of "natural" since there are no artificial products implanted.

If you have an interest in this procedure, you will have to do the research yourself. In their recent position paper on fat grafting: *"The American Society for Aesthetic Plastic Surgery and the American Society of Plastic Surgeons, in the interest of patient safety, do not recommend fat grafting for breast enhancement at this time. Because there is little clinical evidence available to document safety and efficacy, we urge patients to consider the procedure as one undergoing continued evaluation."*

"Natural" Breast Enhancement

It's common, especially in health related journals, to see ads recommending "Natural" Breast enlargement. The ads usually refer to the use of plant-derived hormones that will stimulate breast growth. DON'T USE THEM! By calling themselves "nutritional supplements" they escape the full review of the FDA and safety standards are NOT established. It's a dangerous myth to think that hormones derived from plants are somehow safer. Hormones derived from plants can be very powerful, and like human hormones, rarely have their effect in only one system of the body. Hormones potentially alter the behavior of numerous body functions. A hormone powerful enough to influence the growth of breast tissue is likely to be causing other unknown and uninvestigated changes. It could be many years before an investigator discovers that users of a certain "natural supplement" have a higher incidence of cancer or other diseases.

Breast Reduction (Reduction Mammoplasty)

The term reduction mammoplasty describes a collection of procedures done to reduce the weight, volume, and the problems associated with excessively large breast. They can also be done to improve the appearance of the breasts. There are three basic types of reductions.

Liposuction alone can reduce the volume and size of moderately enlarged breasts, when there is no excess skin that needs to be removed. It can also be the procedure of choice for minor asymmetry. When I'm doing an augmentation mammoplasty on someone with minor to moderate asymmetry, two different size implants will never truly match; remember, height, shape, diameter, volume, and projection will all be different. A simpler solution, is to liposuction a slight amount from the larger breast and then do the augmentation with two of the same size implants. Liposuction is frequently combined with the other reduction techniques when the excess breast tissue extends into the armpit area.

A Pedicle Breast reduction refers to a procedure that moves the nipple areola complex to the desired location on a "pedicle" and then reduces and reshapes the breast to support them in the new position. The pedicle, in addition to the nipple and areola, carries the nerves and blood supply to support them. The pedicle can originate from the top (superior), the bottom (inferior) or from the sides (medial or lateral). This technique is the most commonly used procedure and is used on large or moderate breasts.

Free-nipple Graft reduction is the procedure reserved for massively large breasts unsuitable or too risky for an excessively long pedicle. In this procedure the nipple areola complex is removed while the breast is reduced and reshaped. The nipple areola complex is put back on the new location as a graft. Because its placed as a graft the possibility of a complete loss of the nipple exists. Return of sensation to the nipple is minimal if at all.

Reduction mammoplasty is most often performed for physical complaints such as; neck, shoulder or back pain, skin breakdown and irritation under the breasts, numbness of the hands, shoulder notching, and inability to find and wear an appropriate bras. The social aspects of very large breasts can be equally debilitating. Difficulty finding attractive clothes, inability to participate in sports or athletic events, and difficulty losing weight, are just a few of the problems.

Insurance coverage of the reduction procedure was common in the past. Now the insurance companies have increased the minimal requirements for coverage to something that in some cases would amount to a mastectomy. You will need to check with your surgeon's office, but be aware that the insurance providers will no longer guarantee coverage. Now they review each case individually. If you were promised coverage by the surgeon, do your own homework and call the insurance company yourself, or you could end up with an unexpected large bill.

Our Plastic Surgery Society suggests that the reduction procedure should only be performed on women over the age of 18. An 18-year old is probably finished with the growth of her breasts and is legally able to make her own decisions, and sign her own consent document. By the time a young lady with massive breasts reaches the age of 18 she's missed out on participating in sports and many other school activities. She's developed a habit of minimal exercise (of necessity) and is probably overweight. She may have a lowered sense of self-esteem with her inability to participate in events, the inability to find fashionable clothing, and the overall sense of not fitting in.

I disagree with the position of our society. I carefully explain to the parents and the patient that the chief risk of doing the procedure at an early age is continued growth of the breasts that could require additional surgery. A small price to pay for a life-changing procedure.

Bilateral Reduction Mammoplasty

Physician Fee – N/A

Goal of the procedure

Reducing the size and weight of the breasts, elevating them into a more natural position permitting increased activity and a return to a more normal life. Reduce or eliminate the symptoms of back, neck and shoulder pain.

Alternatives

Special support bras may help with some of the symptoms but not the problem.

Who is a good candidate?

Healthy patients with symptomatic large breasts who can accept the minor imperfections and scarring of the surgery. One of my patients told me; "My goal isn't twins, I'll be happy with sisters!"

Who should avoid?

Unhealthy patients or those who are unable to accept the scarring and surgical results. The pattern of the scarring is usually described as the "inverted T" or "anchor". Patients with high risk of cancer need additional discussion and may choose to modify the procedure.

Operator skill level (1-10) – 6-7

Discomfort (1-10) – 5-8

Anesthesia - General

Length of procedure – 2-4hours

Recovery Time – 3-6 months before the breasts are completely healed and take on the natural round shape. One year for the scars to fully improve.

Return to work – 1-2 weeks

Potential complications
Inconveniences (Level 1)

Drains may be used, swelling, bruising, reduced sensation, and unnatural appearance (flat on bottom edge for several months), difficulty sleeping and shaving armpit.

Difficulties (Level 2)

Bleeding, pain, aseptic fat necrosis[G] (limited non-infectious drainage from the breast), minor wound separation, spitting of the absorbable sutures.

Problems (Level 3)

Loss of the nipple areola complex. (rare even with grafting technique). It can be rebuilt with a combination of tattoo and additional surgery. Loss of pigmentation of all or part of the nipple areola complex (repair with tattoo). Wound separation or breakdown. Malposition of the nipple[PSE] (easy to raise later, nearly impossible to lower)

Description of typical procedure (Inferior Pedicle)

Marking of the breasts is done before going to the operating room. Once in the room, you're given general anesthesia and all the prepping and draping is done. The most important part of the surgery (the pedicle) is addressed first. When finished it will look like the tongue of a shoe with the nipple areola complex (NAC) on the end. The outer layers of skin are removed from the pedicle sparing the NAC. Once the pedicle is completed, wedges of skin and breast tissue are removed medially (center), laterally (near armpit) and superiorly (above). These wedges are carefully weighed for comparison side-to-side and for the goal weight. The breast may be checked for appearance by using a few trial sutures or staples. When satisfied with the new size, position, and symmetry, the temporary sutures are removed and replaced with the permanent sutures. Drains may be placed but are becoming less common. Bulky bandages are applied and you are transferred to the recovery area.

Recovery instructions

Continue to wear the compression stockings for a minimum of 24 hours. Some movement around the house or apartment is encouraged. The first dressing change is usually done in the doctor's office one or two days after the surgery. You will be changed to a bra with light bandages and may begin to shower. Activity is restricted to lifting 15 pounds or less for one week and avoiding bouncy activities for two weeks. You may drive a car when you feel ready but not before two days. You may resume sexual activity after 3-5 days but not "missionary position" for several weeks.

Male Breast Reduction (Gynecomastia)

Young men with excessive breast development suffer just as much as the women. They avoid sports, don't want to take off their shirt, won't go to a pool or a beach and withdraw from any activities that would expose them to teasing. Doctors used to subject them to extensive and expensive hormonal testing but now with no other indicators of hormonal issues, it's rarely done. One theory is that in the early stages of puberty, the first testosterone is made by the adrenal gland and that gland isn't always good at it. The developing body misreads the new hormone as an estrogen and begins to develop a body with female characteristics. By the time the testicles begin producing a better testosterone some minor (and sometimes major) breasts have already formed. Male breasts can also be the result of body building steroids and other medications.

Insurance companies, always looking for ways to deny payment, insist on the patient being close to their ideal weight. This rarely makes a difference.

Severe gynecomastia is uncommon and may require a procedure and scarring similar to a reduction mammoplasty. Most gynecomastia is relatively small (to the surgeon) but huge to the young man who has it. Most commonly, the procedure only requires a small liposuction and a tiny incision to remove a part of the breast button.

Gynecomastia Correction

Physician Fee – $3,051

Goal of the procedure

A normal appearing male chest with a minimum of scarring

Alternatives

None

Who is a good candidate?

Healthy males who are able to reduce their activity for the two required weeks and with a good acceptance of the small amount of scarring.

Men, near or at their ideal weight (especially if submitting to insurance) and completely though puberty.

Who should avoid?

Unhealthy males or males unable to accept the minor differences. All bilateral procedures will have minor asymmetries. A cautious sign is a male seeking a correction of a problem that the doctor can't see. This is another, common presentation of Body Dysmorphic Syndrome[G] and requires psychological counseling NOT surgery.

Operator skill level (1-10) – 5 (this is another procedure which appears simple tempting other surgeons to perform, but in actuality is difficult to do well)

Discomfort (1-10) – 4-5

Anesthesia – General or local with sedation

Length of procedure – 1-2 hours

Recovery Time – The final improvement will take 6 to 8 weeks

Return to work - 2-3 days with restrictions on bouncy activities and restricted weights

Potential complications
Inconveniences (Level 1)
Drains, swelling, bruising, discomfort, difficulty sleeping

Difficulties (Level 2)
Hematoma, bleeding, infection, temporary loss of sensation to the nipples
All patients will have some temporary irregularity, hardness and lumpiness.

Problems (Level 3)
The "Saucer deformity" was the most common problem in general, and is still the most frequent problem in Non-Plastic Surgeon repairs. It represents an over resection of the fatty breast tissue and a depression (saucer) of the chest wall. It can be difficult to repair.[PSE]

Ptosis or sagging of the nipple

Color or tissue loss to the nipple

Unsatisfactory scarring[PSE], prior to the use of liposuction, treatment frequently involved a large chest scar that extended medially (toward the breast bone) and laterally (toward the armpit) and was sometimes more of a deformity than the gynecomastia. (Caution, this is still being done)

Minor recurrences can occur.

Description of typical procedure

After marking, you are taken to the Operating Room and transferred to an OR bed. Anesthesia and local are administered. Two tiny incisions are made in the lower area of the chest. Fluid is introduced into the fatty areas of the breast with a cannula to swell the fat cells and shrink the blood vessels (tumescent fluid[G]). Once the fat cells have swollen, (turgor) liposuction with a very fine cannula is performed matching the volumes from the two sides and being careful not to take too much fat and create the "saucer". A "smile" incision is then made along the lower edge of the areola and a portion of the breast button removed to complete the new contour. A drain is placed through one of the suction incisions and the incision is closed. Light bandages and a compression garment are put in place prior to transfer to the recovery area.

Recovery instructions

Drain care is explained in the office and the recovery area. You may remove the compression garment for showering but then replace it. No heavy lifting or bending. No aerobic or bouncy activities for 3 weeks. Most patients will wear the compression garment for 2 weeks and then change to a tight, stretchy, athletic shirt for an additional 3-4 weeks.

Breast Lift (Mastopexy)

Sagging of the breasts in Plastic Surgery terms is referred to as ptosis[G]. Grades 1 through 4 is used to describe the relationship of the nipple areola complex (NAC) to the inframammary fold or crease. Observed from the side, a Grade I ptosis will have the NAC just at the level of the inframammary fold while a grade 4 will have the entire NAC below the fold. The ligaments that support and anchor the breast onto the chest wall are called Cooper's ligaments. Stretching or weakening of the ligaments can be congenital, from weight gains and losses, children, or exercising without proper support.

Surgery to correct ptosis is called a mastopexy[G] . Although there is promising work outside the US using mesh and other synthetic materials to take the place of the weakened ligaments, these procedures and materials are not approved in the US.

Pseudoptosis or false sagging is commonly seen in women who have breastfed and lost volume while still retaining the ligaments. Although it can look like true ptosis, the difference is the intact ligaments. The solution for pseudoptosis is restoration of volume, and the good news is, it is easily done with implants.

Insertion of ever increasing sizes of implants to compensate for true ptosis is a Fool's Game. Any gain achieved by the large implants is rapidly lost as the added weight of the implants puts traction on the breast and aggravates the ptosis.

Most ptosis correction involves removing a small amount of skin in a pre-planned pattern. The remaining skin is arranged to support the breast in the new and elevated position (sometimes referred to as a dermal bra). The patterns used have different names. Which pattern is chosen is based on the degree of the ptosis and personal preferences.

Types of Ptosis Corrections:

Crescent Mastopexy – Shaped like the crescent moon, this is the smallest mastopexy. It can lift the NAC a full inch or it can shift the NAC medially or laterally.

Periareolar Mastopexy (doughnut) – Although there are Plastic Surgery masters of this technique, for most of us, this is a difficult procedure to get consistent good results. Skin removal is in the shape of a lopsided doughnut. After the initial wound closure, the breast will show puckering around the areola for several months. The puckering eventually corrects itself, but then later if the scar stretches it can form a light ring around the areola similar to the bullseye of a target.

Lollipop Mastopexy – A mastopexy for moderate sagging. The scar pattern resembles a lollipop with a circular incision around the areola and a vertical extension from the areola toward the inframammary fold.

Short Scar Mastopexy – A technique for a larger mastopexy with the usual vertical incision but a small horizontal component in the inframammary crease.

Inverted T Mastopexy – The largest mastopexy for the most severe ptosis. Scars are identical to the breast reduction; around the NAC, vertical and along the inframammary fold making the "T".

Breast Lifts

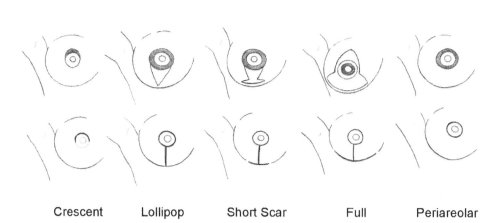

| Crescent | Lollipop | Short Scar | Full | Periareolar |

Mastopexy - Full

Physician Fee - $4,286

Goal of the procedure

The restoration of higher and tighter breasts in a more natural position that is aesthetically appealing and age appropriate.

Alternatives

In clothing, a properly fitting bra can restore position. Out of clothing – none.

Who is a good candidate?

Healthy women, not on blood thinners or serious medications that are able to accept the minor imperfections of the surgery. Patients with asymmetry.

Who should avoid?

Ladies with unrealistic goals or who are overly concerned about the scarring created by these procedures. Women who have more than 15 pounds of planned weight loss. Smokers have increased risk of problems. Patients with high risk of breast cancer need special considerations

Operator skill level (1-10) – 6-8

Discomfort (1-10) - 5

Anesthesia - General

Length of procedure – 2-3 hours

Recovery Time – 3 months for the shape to stabilize

Return to work – a few days to 1 week for smaller procedures, 2 weeks for larger

Potential complications

Inconveniences (Level 1)

Swelling, bruising, difficulty with sleeping, bandages, temporary shape abnormalities with flattening along the lower border of the breast.

Difficulties (Level 2)

Bleeding, wound problems, or numbness

Problems (Level 3)

Malposition of the nipple areola complex[PSE], asymmetry that could require a secondary procedure, depigmentation of the nipple areola, rapid recurrence of the ptosis, permanent numbness, or unsatisfactory scarring

Description of typical procedure

After marking, you're taken to the Operating Room and transferred to the OR bed. Anesthesia and local are administered. The outer layers of the ski are surgically removed in the pattern agreed upon (de-epithelialized[G]). The nipple areola complex (NAC) is shifted to the planned location and the skin repaired to support the breast tissue. Light bandages and a support bra are used.

Recovery instructions

You may change dressings (not the steristrips) as needed. Initially, there will be some minor bleeding on them. You may shower when you feel up to it, just pat the steri's dry and replace a light bandage and bra. Gentle exercise like walking can begin one or two days after the surgery. You may progressively increase your activity but don't begin "bouncy" exercises and aggressive aerobic activities for three weeks.

Bras

Fashion Bras give the least support but the most attractive look and can be used to hold bandages in place and avoid tape. To give any support, they must be fitted carefully and most clerks aren't trained. One of the reasons it's estimated that 50% of American women are wearing the wrong size bra.

Sports Bras are less fashionable but with more support, usually they have a much higher elastic content and the fitting is easier. The level of "Support" can be tested by trying on the bra, gently bouncing up and down while noting the sensation of tugging in the upper part of the breast. The more the sensation of tugging, the less support is being provided by the bra.

Jog Bras were developed for distance runners and stop all movement of the breast. Once you're healed they may be a good choice for very active women. During the healing they have too much pressure and can interfere with the healing.

Congenital Problems Affecting the Breasts

Tuberous Breast[G] – A poorly understood congenital breast deformity. It can be unilateral or bilateral and is characterized by internal bands and constrictions. The shape of the breast is reminiscent of a potato (tuber) with a narrow diameter along most of the length of the breast. Many surgeons and much of our literature suggest treating this with aggressive procedures that lift and/or reshape the breast but leave considerable scarring. I've had good success and minimal scarring with breast implants, the internal release of constricting bands, and PATIENCE. I tell my patients that it may take a full year for all the internal constrictions to release and the breasts to take their final form. If they can be patient, the final result will be aesthetically good and with much less scarring. Be cautious, and do your homework before undergoing unnecessary aggressive surgery.

Poland's Syndrome[G] – A one-sided congenital breast deformity characterized by a muscle defect in addition to an absent or smaller breast. In its most severe form, the syndrome can also have webbed fingers and webbed toes of the affected side. Surgical correction must take into account the reduced or absent muscle with a specially designed implant or a shaped implant. FDA acceptance of the shape-stable cohesive implants will make this correction a lot easier.

Pectus Excavatum[G] – A deformity sometimes referred to as "funnel chest". It consists of a very deep sunken breastbone (sternum) that distorts the appearance of the breasts and gives inward pointing nipples. Simple implants can camouflage some of the problem, mastopexy to move the nipples out laterally can be even more effective and a separate sternal implant or surgery on the sternum is still more effective. In its most severe form, the depressed sternum can interfere with cardiac function and require surgery to change the breast bone.

Scoliosis[G] – refers to a side-to-side curvature of the spine. I mention it here only because women with scoliosis will never be able to achieve perfect breast symmetry. Good but not perfect. Examination for Scloliosis is simple and best identified prior to planned surgery. The degree of scoliosis can be estimated by asking the patient to slowly bend forward while observing the spine from behind.

Trust Me, I'm a Plastic Surgeon

Chapter Ten
The Body

"Your body will tell you what it needs."
--Jennifer Aniston

"If I had known I was going to live this long I would have taken better care of myself."
--Mickey Mantle

Liposuction

Liposuction has become one of the most popular and successful Plastic Surgery procedures. In spite of that, numerous misconceptions and misunderstandings exist about liposuction. The underlying principle is that fat cells have little to no ability to reproduce or grow back once they've been removed. German physicians tried removal with rotating knives on the end of a rod and a weak suction to remove the fat and debris. The procedure worked but caused too much damage. French physicians reversed this with a powerful suction and blunt-edged instruments. They reasoned, correctly, that the fragile fat cells would be damaged and removed by the suction while the more important nerve and vascular tissues would remain intact. And that, girls and boys, was the birth of liposuction.

Facts and Fictions

1. Liposuction **is not** for weight loss. High volume liposuctions can cause fluid shifts and internal bodily changes that can mimic the changes seen with serious burns. Conscientious Plastic Surgeons will limit the amount of fat removed to about 5-7 pounds or about five liters of fluid. Exceeding this can create internal unstable fluid shifts that could require hospitalization and lead to major problems.

2. Liposuction **is** for "problem" areas. With limits on the volumes removed, the procedure is really designed to deal with specific problem areas. A 5-pound fat removal on an obese abdomen would be insignificant while that same 5 pounds on a problem area such as the hips can make an enormous difference.

3. About 70% of the fat **is** physically removed at the time of the procedure, while another 30% is damaged and removed by the body's cleanup mechanism. This later cleanup is a slower process and explains why you will probably be told that the final result may take six months.

4. Removal of the fat creates laxity of the overlying skin. Support garments

must be worn for 4 to 6 weeks to prevent permanent sagging of this skin. The support garments can also help to reduce bruising and swelling.

5. The addition of tumescent solution[G] to the procedure was a major improvement. Injection of large fluid volumes with adrenaline to constrict blood vessels prior to the liposuction, swells the fat cells, reduces bleeding, reduces the risk of irregular surfaces, reduces postoperative fluid requirements and makes the procedure easier to perform for the surgeon.

6. The treated areas are sometimes described as "privileged". These are areas that can easily gain weight but are difficult to lose. In men; the abdomen and love handles are the most common. In women; the abdomen, flanks, inner thighs, hips, saddle-bags, knees, arms and back are all potential areas.

7. It isn't unusual after liposuction that your slacks and dress sizes haven't changed, they just fit better.

8. When I'm asked how much fat I plan to remove? My answer is "I don't know." A surgeon imagines how much fat he / she needs to leave behind for a smooth, attractive figure and then removes the rest.

9. Fat removed by liposuction is not suitable for fat grafting. Typical liposuction settings will rupture the fat cells. Fat for grafting is harvested with a much more gentle technique and lower pressures.

10. Fat cells are not dumb. Evidence now exists that fat cells have the ability to communicate with the rest of the body by chemical messages. The removal of fat cells can even have a dramatic and beneficial effect on some types of diabetes.

11. After weight loss on a crash diet, the least indiscretion can bring the weight loss back with a vengeance. After liposuction, if you maintain the same diet and activity level, the fat will not come back. If you have a dramatic weight gain, some of the gain may distribute to areas that previously weren't problems. There is a story about a famous male singer who had multiple liposuctions in lieu of diet. Previously, he would go on road tours with several sizes of clothes. As the poor traveling diet got to him and the weight gain started, he would just change to a different size. After his multiple liposuctions, his weight gains distributed to other areas.

After several weeks his face had become so round and full he had to cancel the rest of his tour. He even tried (unsuccessfully) to sue his Plastic Surgeon.

12. Liposuction has limited ability to tighten the skin. Every new variation of liposuction claims better skin tightening but none are really that effective. It is dishonest of a Plastic Surgeon to go ahead with liposuction on someone who has excess skin. They know they're going to require a second surgery and a second fee but the patient will end up paying a lot more for the pair of surgeries. Excess skin or skin that has lost its elasticity needs to be removed by one of the tuck procedures.

13. Be cautious of a surgeon who offers you liposuction in his/her office under local anesthesia. This may be acceptable for a modest liposuction, but not for large areas. In large quantities, local anesthetics are NOT safer than general anesthesia. The doctor could be recommending an office procedure because he/she isn't properly trained and cannot get privileges in a certified operating room. The Florida podiatrist doing liposuction in his back room to pay for his child's college is going to tell you it's much safer than going to the hospital with general anesthesia. (Real case! Beware)

Types of Liposuction:

1. Tumescent also called "wet" or "super wet " (used in virtually all procedures)

2. Power Assisted Liposuction (PAL): A motored device that rapidly moves the cannula a small distance in and out. It offers some advantages in control and the speed of the procedure.

3. Ultrasonic: The tip of this device vibrates at a high frequency to emulsify the fat. It shows advantages in a few areas like the back and male breasts that tend to have dense fat, but increases the risk of complications.

4. Laser Liposuction: A laser fiber on the end of a rod. The laser disrupts the fat cells and another suction device carries them away.

5. Water Jet: A newer procedure that floats out the fat cells with high-pressure water. This procedure is gaining interest as fat grafting becomes more popular. Traditional liposuction destroys the fat cells and but the

water jet preserves them for simultaneous use in grafting. Fat cell storage doesn't work.

6. Non–invasive fat removal procedures: They include Cold, Ultrasound, Radio Frequency, Lasers and vitamin injections. Less effective, but less invasive, they can be an alternative to liposuction. They're constantly improving and may be a good choice for small areas. Before agreeing to one of these, find out the usual number of treatments, multiply this by the cost per treatment to be certain you have a good estimate of the total cost. A modest charge for a treatment that needs to be repeated 6 or 8 times can end up far more expensive than you plan. (see more info in the next chapter)

Tumescent Liposuction

Physician Fee - $2,859 (usually per area)

Goal of the procedure

To restore or create a pleasant body contour with balance by the selective removal of fat deposits in problem areas

Alternatives

Diet and exercise.

Who is a good candidate?

People in good health, not on blood thinners, at or near their appropriate weight with one or more problem areas.

Who should avoid?

People with loose and sagging skin, people in poor health or who are seeking large weight reductions in multiple areas. Women on aggressive hormonal therapy or with a history of clots.

Operator skill level (1-10) - 5

Discomfort (1-10) - 5

Anesthesia – General or local with sedation.

Length of procedure – 1-2 hours

Recovery Time – 3-6 months for full recovery

Return to work – 2-3 days if bouncy activities can be avoided.

Potential complications
Inconveniences (Level 1)
Uncomfortable garment, leakage from the entrance wounds (usually the first night only, the drainage can be distinguished from bleeding because its dark pink instead of red and it doesn't clot), swelling, temporary weight gain (don't check)

Difficulties (Level 2)
Infection, hematoma^G , seroma^G , asymmetry, or numbness

Problems (Level 3)
Scarring, over treated depressed areas, surface irregularities or dimples, fat embolism^G, deep venous thrombosis^G (clots), skin loss (especially from ultrasonic), death

Description of typical procedure
Markings are usually done prior to going to the operating room. Once in the OR you would be moved to the operating table and anesthesia administered. Several small puncture incisions are made for access to the areas to be liposuctioned. When possible, two points of access are better for each area. The liposuction cannulas can then crisscross with a reduced risk of surface irregularity.

Tumescent fluid is instilled into the areas to swell the fat cells and shrink the blood vessels. After adequate tissue turgor (swelling) is achieved, liposuction is begun with the appropriate cannulas and technique. Ongoing measurements of total fat removed, as well as side-to-side comparisons are done. When the goal is achieved, the small wounds are closed with dissolving sutures and band-aids. A compression garment is placed to prevent swelling and support the skin.

Recovery instructions

Continue with the support stockings for at least the first full day. Movement (not exercise) for the first day also helps to prevent DVT. Do not shower the day of the surgery but you may the next day. After showering, put the garment back on before additional swelling can occur. Expect some leakage the first night, but if it clots or looks like blood, call the doctor's office. Early moderate activity is encouraged. Bouncy or strenuous activity should be avoided for three weeks. Some type of support garment must be worn for 4-6 weeks.

Notes: Liposuction is frequently combined with other procedures such as breast surgery if you're healthy enough.. The combination, compared to doing them separately, reduces the cost and shortens the recovery time.

Liposuction has been done for patients with Type 2 diabetes. Not only have many of them experienced significant improvement, some have even been cured. Good luck trying to convince your insurance company of this.

Aggressive liposuction (called liposculpting) can be done to define the abdominal muscles (six-pack) by reversing the cannula and suctioning the undersurface of the skin.

Liposuction can be done with the cannula reversed in the armpit to remove most of the sweat glands or to treat a disease called hidradenitis[G].

Abdominoplasty

The tummy tuck or abdominoplasty is used to improve the abdominal area when you have loose sagging skin and loss of elasticity. I frequently hear from women that their husbands don't understand why spending more time at the gym doesn't solve their concerns about their sagging belly. There is no known way to restore the elasticity or to shrink the skin. The only option is removal of the excess skin in an aesthetically acceptable pattern.

In the past there was debate on the combination of liposuction with the surgical incisions of the abdominoplasty. The concern was that the combination could increase the risk of problems. I was at a meeting in Brazil when a brilliant solution was presented, which in my mind makes it the "Brazilian Technique". The concept is simple, liposuction above the umbilicus without cutting, and surgical lifting of the skin below the umbilicus without liposuction. This technique spares the nerves and blood vessels in the upper abdomen while mobilizing the skin just as much as the wider surgical elevation did. Another technical refinement was added by a French Plastic Surgeon who taught us how to minimize the risk of fluid accumulation post-operatively by progressively suturing the skin in place and leaving some lymphatically rich tissues in the lower corners of the abdomen.

Abdominoplasty with Muscle Repair

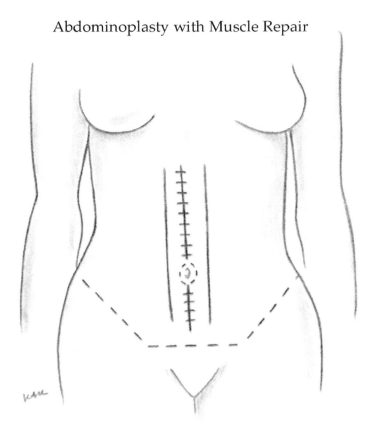

Abdominoplasty

Physician Fee - $5,279

Goal of the procedure

Removal of the excess skin and stretch marks, repair of any muscle separation (diastasis recti[G]) and the restoration of a flat and aesthetically pleasing abdomen.

Alternatives

None

Who is a good candidate?

Healthy people, not planning additional children and anxious to regain some of their pre-baby figure. Not on blood thinners or major medications. People who have had large weight losses and now have excessive skin.

Who should avoid?

Anyone who is still considering additional children or have not waited a full 3 months after the birth of their last child. People who medically cannot tolerate a lengthy surgical procedure. People on blood thinners or medications that interfere with healing.

Operator skill level (1-10) – 5,6

Discomfort (1-10) – 7-9

Anesthesia - General

Length of procedure – 2-4 hours

Recovery Time – 3 months for full aggressive activities and 1 year for final aesthetic result

Return to work – 2 weeks although some work from home is possible before that

Potential complications

Inconveniences (Level 1)

Stockings, compression garment or binder, drains, bruises, swelling, difficulty standing fully erect, muscle cramping, pain and easy fatigue.

If the area just above the pubis is not already numb from a previous C-section, it will be after the abdominoplasty and it's permanent.

Difficulties (Level 2)

Seroma, prolonged need for drains, prolonged difficulty with standing, "dog ears" or small tented up areas at the corners of the incision (repaired in 3 months)

Hernias are frequently encountered and repaired at the time of the abdominoplasty

Problems (Level 3)

Wound problems with delayed healing or separation, infections, skin loss, persistent seroma, umbilical distortion, cannula penetration of the abdomen and the need for emergency intra-abdominal surgery[PSE], DVT with potentially fatal clots

Description of typical procedure

You are marked pre-operatively, moved into the OR and transferred to the OR bed. Anesthesia is administered. A bladder (Foley) catheter is necessary to keep the bladder empty during the procedure. The surgery begins by making several small incisions in the portion of the abdominal skin that will be discarded. Through these incisions tumescent solution is infused to the upper abdomen and the lower outer corners of the abdomen. After adequate tissue turgor, liposuction of the upper abdomen and lower corners is performed.

I begin the surgical part with a "W" shaped incision along the lower abdomen, below any previous C-section scars, and within the bikini line. The

"W" shape allows for more flexibility in adjusting the closure and permits some pull laterally to improve the waist. The incision spares the fibrous tissue in both lateral areas and continues north to the belly button. The umbilicus is detached from the flap and a small tunnel is extended to the upper abdomen. Any muscle separation (diastasis[G]) is repaired both above and below the umbilicus with sutures. The abdominal flap is advanced toward the pubic area. New markings are made with the patient bent slightly. An incision is made to reinsert the umbilicus into the abdominal wall and it's sutured in place. Two drains are placed from the pubic area under the advancing flap. Sutures are placed under the flap to tack it in place and the lower edge is trimmed. Wounds are then closed in three layers with steri-strips to support the skin. Bandages and a compression garment are placed, the drains are activated, and you are ready to be moved to the recovery area.

Recovery instructions

Continue with the support stockings for the first full day at a minimum. Movement (not exercise) for the first day also helps to prevent DVT. Do not shower until the dressings have been changed in the office. Keep records of your drain and bring them to the office. You will need a person to stay with you for the first few days. Someone who could run out to the store, help you get up and down, help to the bathroom and help with any children at home. The first five days after the procedure are the most uncomfortable. We give all our patients narcotics and muscle relaxers. Some prefer the relief from the muscle relaxers over the narcotics.

Expect to have discomfort for the first five days followed by another week of low energy. Drains can usually be removed after five days. After the first dressing change in the office, showers are encouraged but instructions are necessary on how to care for the drains during a shower.

Mini Abdominoplasty

A procedure that sounds better on paper than in real life. Theoretically if the only skin laxity you have is below the umbilicus, then the mini tummy tuck should solve it. I've seen very few women who actually fit those criteria and many more who had the procedure and now complain of; a belly button that is uncomfortable and pulled too low, continued laxity of the skin above the umbilicus, and a bulge in the upper abdomen from the unrepaired muscle separation.

The Ab Paradox

Several years ago after seeing two ladies with the similar situations, I wrote an article for a fitness magazine explaining this paradox. Not wanting to publish any "surgical solutions", they rejected it. The paradox can occur in women with very low body fat, have had several children, and are very fit. They become concerned that their waist is not attractive when they lead or participate in exercise and resolve to increase their activity even more. After a few months of extra crunches and sit-ups, not only is there no improvement, but their waist has begun to get larger (the paradox). The explanation is in the muscles.

When the two strap muscles down the front of the abdomen (rectus muscles) have been separated by pregnancy, they're no longer able to effectively help with crunches or sit-ups. If you persist in doing exercises that require these muscles, the external oblique muscles have to join in to help the ineffective rectus muscles. Continued exercise and use of the external oblique muscles will cause them to grow, like any other muscle. Although the oblique muscles are positioned on the front of the abdomen they extend around the sides or the waist. Increasing muscle mass equals increasing size of the waist. The paradox; the more you exercise to improve your waist, the worse it gets. The only solutions are to stop exercise, or to repair the rectus muscle separation. I did an abdominoplasty on both women and within a year of the surgery they both saw an improvement in their crunches and reductions of their waist sizes

Notes (and some things to look for in photographs)

- It may sound silly but it's important to discuss with your surgeon your concept of an attractive belly button. The ideal shape, and angle of the belly button varies with individual preferences and cultural differences. One nearby surgeon regularly leaves belly buttons the size of ping pong balls. (very difficult to fix!)

- A "T-shape" incision on the lower portion of the abdomen is unsightly and is rarely necessary if the procedure has been designed correctly from the onset.

- Massive weight loss patients will need their drains in much longer than other patients and they are at increased risk for wound complications because of their compromised immune system.

- Doing an abdominoplasty immediately following delivery is dangerous and not recommended by either the Plastic Surgery Societies or the Obstetrical Societies

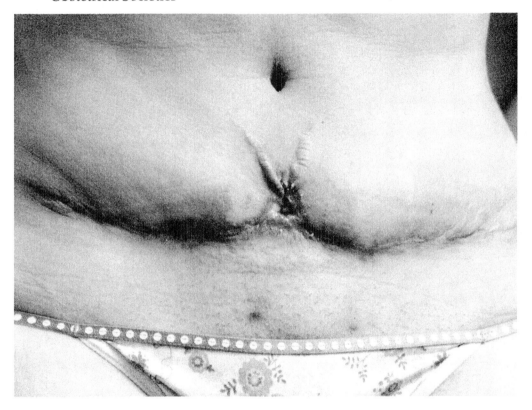

23 yo female with an infected tummy tuck done in South America. It took her five tries to find a Plastic Surgeon who would care for her. She also has very unsatisfactory scars of the breast and the nipples point to the sky.

Arm Lift – Brachioplasty[G]

A Brachioplasty is a procedure done to improve the loose and sagging skin of the upper arms (bat wings) caused by weight loss of aging. Good results are sometimes possible with liposuction alone, but your surgeon will have to make the determination of surgical skin removal vs liposuction.

It's a requirement that all of your rings are removed prior to surgery. Swelling of the hands is possible after the surgery and a tight ring can become dangerous. One of many tricks is to wrap a string tightly around the finger and slip one end under the ring. As you unwind the string, off comes ring. http://www.wikihow.com/Remove-a-Stuck-Ring. If that doesn't work, it's a lot less damaging to the ring to have it removed by a jeweler than an OR nurse.

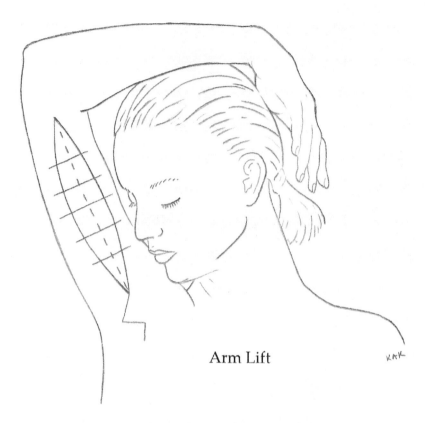

Arm Lift

Brachioplasty (Arm Lift)

Physician Fee[1] - $3,809

Goal of the procedure

The removal of excess flabby skin and fat to reduce and tighten the upper arm.

Alternatives

None

Who is a good candidate?

Persons who are weight stable, not on blood thinners, in good general health and accepting of the large scar from the procedure.

Who should avoid?

Persons who are actively pursuing weight loss, persons on major medications or blood thinners. Persons with edema or poor circulation of the arms. Post mastectomy patients.

Operator skill level (1-10) - 5

Discomfort (1-10) - 5

Anesthesia - General

Length of procedure – 1.5-3 hours

Recovery Time – 3 months until final results, 1 year for optimum scar healing

Return to work - One week, with limitations

Potential complications
Inconveniences (Level 1)

Can be very difficult to keep bandages on the arms, discomfort, swelling of arm or hand.

Difficulties (Level 2)

Numbness, difficulty using the hands, wound separation or delayed healing. A small separation in the arm pit is common and generally heals without problems.

Problems (Level 3)

Major vascular injury[PSE], a surgical emergency requiring a vascular surgeon to come to the OR. A major nerve injury[PSE] (would require repair but not necessarily on an emergency basis). Scarring, skin loss, inability to close the wound[PSE]. (The arm can swell so quickly that a slow surgeon can fall behind and find him/herself unable to close the wound)

Description of typical procedure

Transfer to the Operating Room with markings in place. Move to the OR table and anesthesia is administered. The procedure is begun with a small stab wound near the elbow. Infusion of the tumescent solution followed by liposuction of excess fat. The incision is then made from just above the elbow following the groove on the underside of the arm and ending in the armpit. Once the posterior skin is lifted, it is overlapped and the amount to be resected is determined. This is done at several locations along the incision. Tacking sutures are placed and the remainder of excess skin is resected between the sutures. A small zigzag incision is necessary in the armpit (axilla[G]) to adjust the remaining skin. The wounds are closed in multiple layers with absorbable sutures followed by steri strips, bandages, and elastic wraps. You are transported to the recovery area with your arms elevated on pillows.

Recovery instructions

Keep your arms elevated as much as possible for the first few days. Showering is possible after the first dressing change in the office. No aggressive use of the arms for three weeks. Some oozing will occur the first night because of the liposuction.

Thigh Lift

The thigh lift is a surgical removal of excess lax skin of the inner thigh. Placement of the scar in an inconspicuous place is easy with the abdominoplasty but nearly impossible with the thigh lift. For this reason it has never gained the popularity of the tummy tuck. Earlier procedures used an incision down the inside or inner (medial) part of the upper leg similar to the arm lift. Obviously, this was a highly visible and unattractive scar location. The procedure evolved to a scar that follows the crease through the crotch from mid-leg in front to mid-buttock crease in the rear. This surgery gives an excellent scar that is well hidden even with a bathing suit, but the excellent results last for only a few years. Although the tightening of the upper leg persists, the scar eventually drifts down the leg and becomes visible when wearing a bathing suit. Different anchoring techniques have been proposed without much success. Who knows? Someone may solve this in the near future.

The procedure can be combined with the abdominoplasty. Judge for yourself, but to my eye the scarring from this combined procedure is unattractive and distinctly unsexy. I never combine the thigh and abdomen since doing them separate gives more options and better scarring.

Thigh Lift

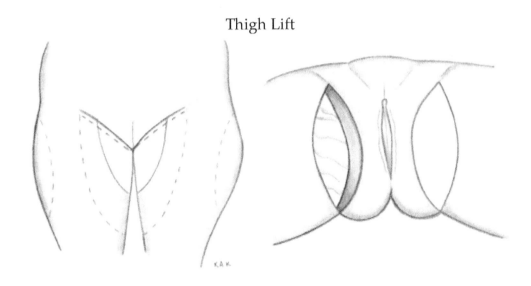

Thigh Lift

Physician Fee[1] - $4,694

Goal of the procedure
The goal is to create a tighter and shapelier upper leg by removal of loose saggy skin and with the least visible scar.

Alternatives
None

Who is a good candidate?

People who have a stable weight within 15 pounds of their goal. Medically fit, not on blood thinners and accepting of the final scars.

Who should avoid?

People with significant medical issues or unable to accept the scarring

Operator skill level (1-10) – 5-6

Discomfort (1-10) – 7-8

Anesthesia - General

Length of procedure – 2-3 hours

Recovery Time – Wounds should be healed within one month. Final healing is one year.

Return to work – 2 weeks

Potential complications

Inconveniences (Level 1)

Initial bandages are difficult to maintain in that area and need frequent replacement, discomfort with sitting or lying down, bruising, swelling

Difficulties (Level 2)

Minor wound problems with irritation or slight separation are common with this procedure. Some may even turn into infection. Tightness or swelling of the area.

Temporary numbness.

Problems (Level 3)

The risk of DVT[G] and clots is a concern with the limited mobility. Permanent numbness[PSE] of small or large areas of the thigh, interference with walking from tightness and pulling, over-correction[PSE] with excessive tension in the vulva area and painful sex. Major vascular or nerve injuries[PSE] requiring emergency surgery.

Description of typical procedure

You would be transported to the operating room with markings in place, transferred to the OR table and anesthesia administered. A foley catheter would be placed and your legs elevated in stirrups. The incision is made from front to rear and leg flap elevated and undermined. Similar to the arms, the incision is overlapped by the leg flap and marking sutures are placed. When all of the marking sutures are in place the intervening skin is removed and the wounds are closed. The key sutures attach the skin to the deeper ligaments of the thigh WITHOUT putting tension on the vulva. Three layers of closure followed by steri strips with bandages. Transfer to the recovery area.

Recovery instructions

Stockings must remain in place for at least the first few days. Walking around a little and bending and flexing of the feet are necessary for DVT[G] protection. Some bleeding or oozing will occur during the first day. You can shower after the first day, just pat the steri strips dry and try to keep a bandage on for the first few days. No serious physical activity or sex for a minimum of three weeks.

Buttock Lift

There are three different buttock lifts and they are sometimes combined with an abdominoplasty or thigh lift. Combined procedures usually require more than one surgeon and a hospitalization of at least a day or two.

The first lift is in the pattern of a belt along the upper portion of the buttocks, which pulls the buttocks toward the area where the belt would be. The second removes an ellipse of skin from the mid-portion of the buttock. It gives a satisfactory lift but leaves a scar which looks like a permanent panty line angling across the buttock. The third removes an ellipse of skin from the lower crease of the buttock and resembles the natural buttock crease when it heals. The third lift can also be used to enhance or augment the buttock by folding the fatty tissue into the incision instead of discarding it.

Butt Lifts

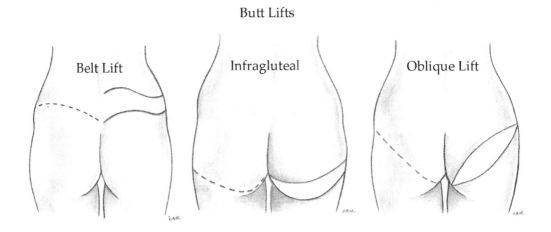

Buttock Lift (gluteal fold technique)

Physician Fee - $4,694

Goal of the procedure
The goal is to lift and reshape the buttocks to a more flattering aesthetic appearance.

Alternatives
Buttock implants (silicone) or fat grafting to increase the size of the buttock if the required lift is minimal. Selective liposuction can reshape the buttocks to a more attractive appearance.

Who is a good candidate?
Those who are medically fit, not on blood thinners or major medications, with a stable weight and accepting of the scars.

Who should avoid?
Those who are overly concerned about the scarring or who are interested in a large volume increase.

Operator skill level (1-10) – 5,6

Discomfort (1-10) – 7-8

Anesthesia - General

Length of procedure – 2-3 hours

Recovery Time – 6 months to fully stabilize.

Return to work – 2 weeks with restrictions

Potential complications

Inconveniences (Level 1)
Swelling, bruising, difficulty sitting, minor bleeding or oozing for the first day

Difficulties (Level 2)
Minor infections, bleeding or temporary numbness

Problems (Level 3)
Wound separation, scarring, asymmetry[PSE]

Description of typical procedure (lower buttock crease with augmentation)
You would be marked before going to the Operating Room. Anesthesia is administered and you are rolled face down (prone) and transferred to the operating table.

Surgery is begun by outlining the skin paddle that will give the lift and be the filler flap. The outer layers of the skin are removed from the paddle (deepithelialized). A pocket is created superiorly to fit the flap. The flap is inserted into the pocket, and trimmed or modified for the precise "look" planned. Sutures are placed in the pocket to prevent shifting or movement of the flap. A drain is inserted and the wound closed in multiple layers. Bandages are applied. You would be rolled back onto a transport gurney and taken to the recovery area.

Recovery instructions

Stockings must remain in place for at least the first few days. Walking around along with bending and flexing of the feet are necessary for DVT[G] protection. Some bleeding or oozing will occur during the first day. You can shower after the first day, just pat the steri strips dry and try to keep a bandage on for the first few days. Limit sitting as much as possible. No strenuous exercise or sex.

Cosmetic Gynecology

The surgery is done to correct the position, shape and volume of the labia majora[G] , the labia minora[G] and the mons pubis[G] for both aesthetic and functional improvements. The increasing popularity of these procedures is thought to derive from the additional exposure shaving provides. Alternatively, the influence of the porn industry on the aesthetics of the area is another possible reason.

The **mons pubis** can become deflated with aging. Without this fatty protection overlying the pubic bone, sex can become uncomfortable or painful. Conversely, the mons area can develop unsightly bulging after a large weight gain. Later, even after losing the weight, some areas don't reduce and the mons can be one of those areas. Surgical correction either adds fat by grafting to inflate the mons or removes fat with liposuction to reduce the mons. Either procedure can be done in the office with just local anesthesia.

The **labia majora** can deflate in the aging process or become asymmetrical. Again, fat grafting can restore balance, symmetry, aesthetic and padding with a simple office procedure and local anesthesia. Excessively large labia majora are easily reduced surgically.

The **labia minora** can become stretched by childbirth or misshapen congenitally. Correction can be done as an office procedure with local anesthesia. A portion of the labia is surgically resected in a pattern that hides the scars and reduces risk of later discomfort. Caution, newer patterns of labia minora reduction are much less likely to cause "notching" or the uncomfortable scars of older procedures.

Laser reshaping of the **vagina** for improved sexual enjoyment has been strongly promoted on the west coast but remains controversial. Studies done and reviewed by the Gynecology associations fail to show the claimed improvement while documenting the added risks of scarring and discomfort. These procedures are not recommended at this time. Consider carefully before undergoing these techniques.

Some Gynecologists are quite skilled in these procedures (you still have to ask; how often they do them, training, and complications). Although less commonly performed by Plastic Surgeons, as demand increases, you can expect more of them will learn these techniques. As always, do your research when choosing your surgeon.

Female Genitalia

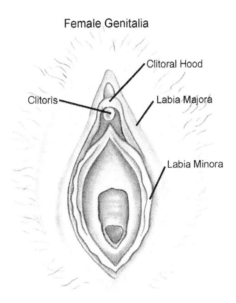

Cosmetic Gynecology

Physician Fee[1] – N/A

Goal of the procedure

The restoration or creation of a younger, balanced and more aesthetic relationship of the three areas.

Alternatives

Fillers can be used as an alternative to fat grafting in deflated areas

Who is a good candidate?

Healthy patients with physiologic or aesthetic problems with one or more of the areas

Who should avoid?

These procedures have the danger of becoming "fads". Make certain of your motivation before having a consultation and only work with a doctor that is fully aware of your goals.

Operator skill level (1-10) - 5

Discomfort (1-10) – 5-6

Anesthesia - Local

Length of procedure – 30 minutes to 1 hour

Return to work – 1 week

Potential complications
Inconveniences (Level 1)

Discomfort, swelling, bruising

Difficulties (Level 2)

Difficulty with urination

Problems (Level 3)

Painful sex with a poorly designed procedure[PSE], scarring, asymmetry[PSE,] scarring that involves the clitoris or the hood of the clitoris can be painful[PSE]

Recovery instructions

Ice compresses intermittently to the area, cleansing and application of antibiotic ointment, restricted sports activity (including sex) for 3 weeks.

Massive Weight Loss Patients

With the increasing use of endoscopic surgery, the number of massive weight loss patients has dramatically increased. The procedures to alter the stomach or the digestive pathway are now safer and more effective. Questions still remains about the long-term effects on the body and the body's immune system, but the long-term effects of morbid obesity on the heart, blood pressure, risk of diabetes, stroke, and joints are well documented.

Plastic Surgeons are seeing increasing numbers of patients who've lost massive amount of weight and want improvement of the loose and sagging skin that remains. The corrective procedures are the same as the ones just described but on a different scale. In a small group practice or a solo practices, these corrections have to be done in stages. For example; surgery of the breasts and abdomen at one time, the thighs another time, and the back and buttocks at yet another time. The advantages include; local care with a trusted surgeon, minimal time off of work, and reduced cost. The disadvantage is the longer period of time before all the surgery is completed. In my experience many of the weight loss patients don't complete all of the possible surgical solutions and are satisfied with an improved abdomen, chest, and arms.

At some of the larger medical centers, Plastic Surgery departments with a special interest in massive weight loss patients can offer larger and more complex combined procedures dealing with multiple areas at the same time. These procedures require multiple surgeons working at the same time and usually several days of hospitalization. For those who are impatient and can afford it, it may be right solution. Researching these programs can be very difficult. I've been to a scientific program where very distinguished surgical groups proudly displayed their results that I (and others in the audience) thought they were so bad that we could barely look at them. I've been to other programs where the results were so stunning, I thought that they were raising the bar for all of the rest of us. I'm sure you're tired of hearing it, but, do your homework, don't fall for the "experts", trust your intuition and I'll add, look at a lot of pictures. If the pictures don't look natural or even human, keep looking, good programs are out there.

Chapter Eleven
The Unusual

"We are in the process of creating what deserves to be called the idiot culture.
Not an idiot sub-culture, which every society has bubbling beneath the surface and
which can provide harmless fun; but the culture itself.
For the first time, the weird and the stupid and the coarse are becoming our cultural
norm, even our cultural ideal."
--Carl Bernstein

This is a collection of some fad surgeries, which could become the Plastic Surgery staples of the future, or they could just disappear.

The FDA requires both proof of safety and proof of effectiveness for approval, but the proof of effectiveness may not be as significant as the manufacturers would have you believe.

Elbow Lift

This is an unusual and rarely requested procedure because of the scarring. It is usually done under local anesthesia. A patch of skin is removed from the area adjacent to or over the mid-portion of the elbow, leaving a permanent scar just above the elbow. During the healing for two to three weeks, only limited bending of the arm is permitted. If it is done too aggressively a permanent restriction of movement can result. One arm is usually done at a time in order to have some ability to care for yourself.

The surgery can be done on a smaller scale with the removal of only a small amount of skin, but the scar is the same.

Complicatons – Not only do you risk permanently restricting motion of the elbow, but a painful, unsightly scar can occur. Hypothetically, which would be more noticeable, a little sagging skin or the scar?

Knee Lift

An identical procedure to the elbow but done on the knee. If you were to ask a Plastic Surgeon "where does a person have the highest risk of bad scars?" The answer would likely be; first over the breastbone and second near a major joint. Bad scar vs. sagging skin again.

Knee and Ankle Liposuction

Not really that unusual in terms of "strangeness" but not frequently done. A small percentage of the population has well defined fat pads either on the medial side of the knee that annoyingly brush against each other when they walk or on the medial side of the ankles. If you have one of these problems, you can have an excellent improvement with a tiny liposuction to these areas. The procedure would probably be done in an office setting with local anesthesia. Ice, elevation and elastic wraps will help reduce and control the swelling and bruising.

Toe Shortening

This is an interesting procedure that has come in vogue on the West coast. (Have you ever wondered why everything weird seems to start on the West coast? Could it be proximity of Mt. Shasta?) The procedure is designed for women who would like to wear open-toed shoes but are self-conscious about a second toe that is longer than the big toe. They feel that this foot arrangement is aesthetically unacceptable and ask surgeons to shorten the offending toe. Understand, this procedure entails a cut (and scar) into the toe, removal of a section of bone and stabilizing the surgical fracture with one or more metal pins that later have to be removed.

Complications - Not only does this procedure have the potential for scars and infection, but this is a real fracture with a minimum of six weeks to heal and the possibility of non-healing. An infection that spreads into the bone can be a difficult and lengthy problem to treat, and can result in loss of the toe. All, in order to wear more stylish shoes.

Cell Phone Neck

People who spend a lot of time on their cell phones have noticed that the usual position of their head on the cell phone camera exaggerates the folds and creases of the neck.("cell-phone neck") They have begun to request either neck lifts and/or chin implants to improve the appearance of the neck on camera. Good results are easily obtained with the standard surgeries.

Dimple Plasty

This is another fad. In an effort to enhance their appearance, especially for males, patients are requesting the creation of dimples in either the cheeks or the central area of the chin, a la Kirk Douglas.

The chin can be easily done in the office with local anesthesia. The cheek is more problematic. If this is a procedure that appeals to you, make certain your doctor has experience and fully appreciates the anatomy. In the area of an ideal cheek dimple, there are multiple very tiny nerves and important muscles that are easily damaged. Inadvertent damage could result in partial paralysis of the face or facial asymmetry.

Mesotherapy

A procedure that is not FDA approved and, in fact, banned in several countries. It consists of micro-injections of a vitamin mixture in a grid pattern over the area with the problem fat. The injections send a chemical message to the fat cells to reduce their size. Effective for small areas, it's only a temporary improvement since it doesn't damage the fat cells and they can always refill. The procedure began in France, was popular in Europe, had a brief enthusiasm in the U.S., but has now waned.

Non-Surgical Techniques

Many of these devices show promise but are far from being universally accepted. In general, the Plastic Surgery societies recommend caution. Some of these non-surgical procedures can hurt you. A few appropriate questions: Who's running the machine?, Where's the doctor who is supposed to be supervising? Do you get to talk to a doctor or just a technician? How many treatments will it take to see the desired result? Can you talk to former patients? Don't forget to bring your intuition. I know it's hard, but when you're doing your research, try to get information that wasn't written by the manufacturer or their paid doctors.

Radiofrequency Fat Ablation

Not yet FDA approved for fat reduction, Dermatologists commonly use it. The radiofrequency energy heats the fat cells without disturbing the skin and destroys them. The manufacturers claim it can be used on any part of the body and has no recovery time.

Ultrasound

Not yet approved by the FDA for fat reduction. The ultrasound from several heads pass harmlessly through the skin and focus on the fat cells. The ultrasound energy causes leakage of the fat cell contents and cell destruction. The technique allows for treatment of large areas but it can be difficult to control and predict the final result.

Cryolipolysis (Cold fat ablation)

One of the newer techniques, which is approved by the FDA. Based on the principle that fat cells are more vulnerable to cold than other tissues, it's used on the lower abdomen and sides. Large areas can be treated but the final results are slow, sometimes taking as long as 6 months.

The company claims they got the idea from observing that children who ate a lot of popsicles had thinner cheeks.

Low Level Laser Fat Ablation (Cold Laser)

An FDA approved low-level laser for fat removal. The laser is programmed to make multiple passes over the area to be reduced. The laser, which is virtually painless, damages the underlying fat cells by causing them to leak. Multiple and frequent treatments are the biggest drawback.

Thread Lifts

This is another category of fads that seem to come and go. The appeal is universal; A facial rejuvenation done in an office with only local anesthesia, minimal expense, no down time, minimal swelling and no discomfort. There are several variations that appear to deliver most of this. The problem is that they have very unpredictable durability, anywhere from a few months to a year or two, at best. Two American lifts used barbed threads or cones to support the lift. One didn't last very long and the other sometimes caused scarring visible through the facial skin. Both were anchored to the deep facial structures at one end of the thread. A Russian (actually Georgian) barbed thread version with wide acceptance all over Europe doesn't anchor the thread at either end. The inventors of this thread claim that the anchoring is the chief reason for the premature failure of most thread lifts.

A newer American version, specific for the neck, crisscrosses the neck in a spider web pattern for a pure neck lift. It is effective, doesn't have an anchor, and is done in an office setting. It remains to be seen how long it will last.

Stay skeptical if you're considering any of these procedures and try to get information on their actual cost and their longevity. Even better, talk to some of the previous patients.

Trust Me, I'm a Plastic Surgeon

Glossary

-ectomy – to remove something surgically

-otomy – to surgically create a hole or an incision

-plasty – Molding or forming surgically

Abdominoplasty – Plastic Surgical correction of loose and sagging abdominal skin frequently with tightening of the abdominal muscles

ABMS – Certifying board for the 24 approved medical specialties

Abscess – localized collection of pus

Acellular Dermal Matrix (ADM) - Processed animal or human skin that has been treated to remove the outer layers of the skin (epidermis) and the cellular elements that would cause rejection or allergy. What remains is an intact matrix of natural biological components that lends strength, becomes vascularized and is incorporated into the skin of the recipient.

Acne vulgaris – One of the most common skin diseases characterized by comedones, and pustular nodules most commonly on the back, chest and face.

Acne rosacea – a type of acne which is characterized by redness and swelling of the face, forehead, cheeks, and nose

Acne scars – the scarring left behind after the acute inflammation of the acne has subsided. They can vary from the small punched out scars (ice pick scars), to large depressed areas to raised red nodules.

Acupuncture – A traditional Chinese discipline which uses needles inserted along meridians to treat symptoms or diseases.

Acute – Immediate or urgent

Adenopathy – Swollen glands (usually lymphatic)

Aesthetic – Artistic, used to describe cosmetic surgery.

Adipose – Fat tissue

Adipocyte – Individual fat cell

Air Hunger – the sensation that you're unable to inhale sufficient air. It may be caused by a surgical alteration of an internal area of the nose called the "Internal Nasal Valve". Repairable.

Alopecia – Loss of hair from an area which normally has it

Anaphylaxis - An acute hypersensitivity (allergic) reaction due to exposure to anantigen. The reaction may include rapidly progressing hives, respiratory distress, vascular collapse, systemic shock and death.

Anesthesia - A state characterized by loss of feeling or sensation. This is usually the result of pharmacologic action to allow performance of surgery or other painful procedures.

Anesthetist – A nurse with special training in the administration of anesthetics

Anesthesiologist – A doctor specializing in the use of anesthetics

Antiemetic – an agent that will prevent or arrest vomiting

Aponeurosis – a fibrous sheet of connective tissue which serves to attach muscle to bone or other tissues.

Arcus Marginalis – A membrane of the lower eyelid which attaches to the orbital rim and holds the orbital fat pads in place.

Areola – A ring like discoloration as around the nipple

Arnica – Homeopathic medication used to reduce bruising. Pill or cream (cream should not be applied to open or fresh incisions)

ASAPS – The American Society of Aesthetic Plastic Surgery
http://www.surgery.org

Aseptic fat necrosis – Occurs most frequently in breast reduction surgery when an area of fat within the breast has compromised blood supply and liquefies. It will drain from the breast as a clear and odorless liquid.

ASPS – American Society of Plastic Surgeons (approved by ABMS)
http://www.plasticsurgery.org

Arm lift – surgical procedure to remove the excess skin (bat wings) of the upper arm. Generally, with a linear incision in the groove of the underside of the arm.

Augmentation – Plastic Surgery which adds or implants something in the body

Axilla – Armpit

Basal cell carcinoma – the most common of the skin cancers, rarely metastasizes or kills but can be quite problematic when it is near an opening to a deeper space such as the nose, ears, or eyes

Biofilm – an aggregation of bacterial cells on the surface of an implanted device. Implicated in heart valve failure, artificial joint failure and breast implant capsular contracture.

Blepharoplasty – a Plastic Surgery operation on the eyelids to remove excess skin and muscle with removal or redistribution of the orbital fat.

Blepharoptosis – Drooping of the upper eyelid

BMI – Body mass index, a calculated measure of body fat that give an indication of nutritional status.

Body Dysmorphic disorder – A psychological illness involving an obsessive fixation with a physical defect either small or imagined to the point it interferes with their life.

Botox® – Medication which is injected into small muscles to temporarily cause relaxation by blocking the nerve impulse. May also be used to reduce other neural activity such as sweating. (Myoblock®, Dysport®)

Bottoming Out – A shift in the mass of the breast or the breast implant into the lower pole of the breast with simultaneous unnatural upward elevation of the nipples. (star gaxers)

Brow Lift – Plastic Surgical procedure to elevate the eyebrows and reduce wrinkles of the forehead (usually done with small incisions and a scope) "endoscopic"

Canthus – The angle formed at the inner and outer corners of the eye

Canthoplasty – A surgical procedure which lengthens the distance between canthi or changes the angle of the outside attachment of the canthus.

Capsule – A thin fibrous sac enveloping an implant usually breast.

Capsulotomy – A surgical incision which cuts a capsule

Capsulectomy – A surgical removal of a capsule.

Capsular Contracture – The most common complications of breast augmentation which can occur weeks to years after an augmentation procedure. It is characterized by scar tissue forming around the implant and resultant hardness, elevation, and discomfort of the affected breast.

Cellulite – Dimpling of the skin overlying an area of fatty deposits probably due to the compartmentalization of the fat, almost exclusively in women

Cellulitis – A spreading bacterial skin infection just beneath the surface

Chemical Peel – The use of strong chemicals to create a controlled skin injury removing the outer layers and improving the appearance. (Blue Peel, ViPeel, phenol, TCA, Croton oil, etc.)

Chin Implant – see *Mentoplasty*

Collagen – A structural component of the skin, bone, ligaments and cartilage and an essential contributor to healing.

Columella – The strip of skin running from the tip of the nose to the lip, separating the nostrils

Concha – The word means shell shaped, usually refers to the deep shell shaped portion of the ear.

Cribriform plate – A fragile bony separation of the upper nose from the brain which can be injured in surgery or trauma.

Crow's Feet – Fine radiating lines at the outer corner of the eyes commonly treated with Botox-like substances.

Deepithelialize – A surgical removal of the outer layers of the skin. Done when the deepithelialized skin is going to be relocated beneath intact skin such as breast reduction or lift.

Deep venous thrombosis – A condition in which one or more clots form in a deep vein, often in the legs. The clots (thrombi) can move to the lungs resulting in death.

Dermabrasion – A mechanical removal or sanding of the outer layers of the skin with a rotating wire brush or sanding wheel. This stimulates healing, improves appearance and reduces irregularities and imperfections

Dermis – The living middle layer of the skin

Diastasis recti – A separation of the two strap muscles of the abdomen usually caused by child bearing. It can interfere with exercise and create an unsightly bulge in the center of the abdomen.

Dog-ear – A tenting up of the ends of a surgical closure which may require a revision

Dry eye – A condition of inadequate tear lubrication of the eye. Following eyelid surgery is usually temporary.

Ectropion – A complication of blepharoplasty in which the lower eyelid separates from the globe and roll outward.

Edema – Swelling caused by excess fluids, usually in the tissues

Endoscopic Brow Lift – See *Brow Lift*

Erythema – Redness of the skin caused by dilation of the capillaries

Eyelid lift – see *blepharoplasty*

Facial Implants – Plastic Surgical procedure to augment a portion of the face. The incision is frequently in the mouth. Types include; Malar, Submalar, Orbital, Nasal and Tear Trough.

Fascia – A sheet of loose connective tissue beneath the skin, which offers structural support and is useful in some lifts for durability (face, midface, neck).

Fat Embolism – Fat globules which block the circulation. Very rare with liposuction but not rare with certain leg fractures

Filler – A substance (natural or artificial) used to elevate or lift a depression of the skin by injecting into or beneath the skin. Commonly used to elevate creases, grooves or depressions of the face.

Flap – Tissue elevated from one part of the body and moved to a different area while maintaining its own blood supply. Usually skin, or muscle, or fat. If the blood supply is reconnected in the new location it is called a "free flap"

Forehead Lift – see *Brow lift*

Frown Lines – see *Glabella*

Fraxel Laser – A Laser with a rapid recovery that works by creating numerous small holes in the skin. After healing the skin has a better texture and appearance.

Frown Lines – One or more vertical lines between the brows (glabella) which are commonly treated with Botox-like substances.

Genioplasty – An operation performed to reshape the chin

Glabella – An area of the forehead between the brows and at the start of the nose. The first area approved for the use of Botox®.

Gynecomastia – Excess development of breasts in male.

Headlights – An unnatural forward facing of the nipples usually caused by the shift of the implants laterally under the arms.

Hemangioma – A benign skin tumor composed of abnormal blood vessels.

Hematoma – A collection of blood usually after a surgical procedure. May be gel at first and slowly turn liquid.

Hidradenitis suppurativa – An inflammatory and infectious disease of the apocrine sweat gland of the armpit or other areas which can result in frequent abscesses and scarring.

Hyperhydrosis – A condition of excessive sweating. It can be a debilitating problem when it occurs in the palms or the soles of the feet.

Hypertrophic Scar – A raised and red scar which is not healing normally. May require an additional procedure to correct.

Internal Nasal Valve – An area of the nose that senses airflow.

Keloid – A genetic wound healing disease in which the body fails to recognize that healing is complete and continues the manufacture of collagen. By definition, a keloid is a scar that exceeds the bounds of the original injury.

Labia majora – The outer fatty folds of the vulva.

Labia minora – The thinner inner folds of the vulva.

Libioplasty – A surgical modification of the lips, or the labia majora

Laser Resurfacing – Laser removal of the outer skin layers creating a controlled burn which heals with an improved surface, reduced wrinkles, birthmarks or scars.

Lip augmentation – Surgical enhancement of the lips can be done with fat, fillers, or an implantable device.

Local anesthetic – an agent which will deaden nerves when applied directly to the skin or mucous membranes or injected.

Lymphedema – A swelling of the subcutaneous tissues due to a blockage of the lymphatic tissues, sometimes surgical.

Liposuction – Surgical removal of fatty tissue using cannulas through small incisions.

Lip Augmentation – A procedure used to fill, enlarge, or define deflated lips. It can be done with surgery, a surgical implant or fillers.

Lipoplasty – Same as liposuction

Lipostructure – Surgical removal of healthy fat, concentration, and used as a filler in various parts of the body.

MACS Lift – A type of mini facelift with a reduced incision, Plication of the SMAS tissues, and a very vertical (anti-gravity) lift.

Marionette lines – An age related skin fold from the corner of the mouth to the edge of the jaw bone.

Mastopexy – Surgical lifting of the sagging breast.

Maxilla – The upper jaw.

Mesotherapy – Injection of high concentration vitamins in a grid pattern to signal the fat cells to shed fatty material. Banned in several countries and not well accepted.

Melanocyte – The pigment cells of the skin which can be damaged surgically, by freezing or by lasers.

Milia –A small white or yellow fluid collection just beneath the skin caused by blockage of the sebaceous glands.

Mondor disease – Phlebitis of a vein of the breast usually after a surgical procedure. Characterized by a linear area of tenderness on the lower portion of the breast. Not dangerous.

Mentoplasty – A surgical alteration of the chin either by modification of the bone (mandible), or by placement of an implant. Used to change facial balance.

Microdermabrasion – A micro "sandblasting" of the outer layers of the skin for a freshening look. It is much less invasive than full dermabrasion.

Mini Tummy Tuck – Removal of a small area of skin below the umbilicus to tighten the skin.

Mons Pubis – a rounded mound of fatty tissue sitting on the pubic bone.

Munchausen syndrome – characterized by repeated fabrication of symptoms and complaints in order to obtain additional surgery.

Nasolabial fold – The two skin folds that run from the corner of the nose to the corner of the mouth.

Necrosis – Death of cells from trauma or disease.

Nipple areola complex – The colored disc of breast tissue including the nipple

Otoplasty – A surgical procedure of the outer ear, usually pinning.

Off-Label – After the approval by the FDA of a therapeutic agent, they do not have the legal authority to regulate the practice of medicine. Under the concept of 'off-label', a physician can legally use the approved drug for an unapproved indication, location, dosage or age. The patient must be informed of off-label usage.

Pectus excavatum – Called "funnel chest" it is a deformity with a sunken or depressed chest bone (sternum). In its severe form the chest bone may interfere with the function of the heart and need urgent surgical correction. In lesser forms it causes a chest and breast deformity.

Poland's Syndrome – A rare birth defect characterized in its minimal form with a small or absent breast on one side and a partial muscle defect. In its full form, the breast is absent, the muscle (pectoralis major) is absent and there can be webbing of the fingers and toes on the same side.

Ptosis – Drooping, (eyelids, breasts, arm skin, thigh skin, abdomen, etc.)

Seroma – A collection of blister fluid (serum)

Scoliosis – a side-to-side curvature of the spine.

SMAS – Superficial Muscular Aponeurotic System – Also called the third layer of the face after skin and fat. In the neck it's a muscle but turns in a fibrous sheet in the face. Used by Plastic Surgeons to enhance and add durability to a facelift.

Smoker's Lines – see *rhagades*

Squamous cell carcinoma – A type of skin cancer arising from the "squamous" portion of the skin. Can be aggressive under certain circumstances

Standing wrinkles – Wrinkles that don't smooth out even when the underlying muscle relaxes.

Symmastia – A problem with breast augmentation that occurs when the implants meet in the middle of the chest to form a single breast (monoboob) with each nipple pointing to the side.

Rhagades – The small vertical lines radiating from the lips (smoker's lines). They can be treated with injections, dermabrasion or laser.

Tuberous Breast – A development disorder of the breast affecting about 1 in 200 women. It is recognized by the presence of internal bands or constrictions shaping the breast into something resembling a potato (tuber).

Tumescent Solution – Saline solution injected directly into tissues to be liposuctioned. Used to swell the fat cells and constrict the small blood vessels. The solution may contain adrenalin and spreading agents.

Tummy Tuck – see Abdominoplasty

Telangiectasia – Chronic dilation of groups of capillaries giving the skin a blush

Telephone ear deformity – A post-surgical ear deformity with protrusion of the upper and lower parts of the external ear and a depressed center.

Temporalis fascia – A strong fibrous layer present in the temple areas of the face used in many suspension procedures.

Thigh lift – A surgical procedure which tightens the loose and saggy skin of the upper thigh.

Thigh-buttock lift – A surgical procedure which tightens loose and saggy skin of both the upper thigh and the buttocks.

Thrombosis – The formation of a clot.

DVT – Deep Venous Thrombophlebitis, clot formation and inflammation of the deep veins of the legs. A very dangerous complications of a surgical

Tissue expansion – A surgical method of inducing the body to grow new skin. Generally by placing and slowly filling a balloon like device beneath the skin.

Torticollis – Wryneck – a spasm of neck muscle in children which causes a twisting and tilt of the head and discomfort.

Tragus – The small bump guarding the entrance to the ear canal. It can be significantly distorted by an inexpert facelift.

TRAM – A breast reconstructive technique using the skin and muscle of the abdomen to create a breast after mastectomy.

Toxic shock syndrome – A potentially fatal rapidly progressive bacterial illness frequently initiated by a retained foreign body such as a nasal packing or other packing

Witch's chin deformity – A cosmetic deformity of the chin with an overhanging portion of the chin and a prominent crease beneath the chin.

W-plasty – A surgical procedure which adds angles to a surgical closure to prevent a linear contracture.

Z-plasty – A Plastic Surgical procedure which alters the length of a scar in two directions to change its tension or direction.

Zygoma – The area of the cheek formed by the zygoma bone and arch.

Appendix

INTUITION
intuition | ˌint(y)oōˈiSHən |
noun
the ability to understand something immediately, without the need for conscious reasoning.
• *a thing that one knows or considers likely from instinctive feeling rather than conscious reasoning.*

Intuition
is not magic, it's not the "force" of Star Wars, it's comes from real data gathered by your brain when the other parts of your brain are too busy living your life.

If someone were to ask you how you make a decision. You would probable answer that you make a decision by listing the pros and cons (mentally or on a sheet of paper) and whichever side of the list has the most compelling entries becomes the decision. That sounds good and, in fact, sometimes that's exactly what you do. Most of the time, however, you make decisions so effortlessly that you don't even realize that you do it. These are the intuitive or "gut" decisions. Decisions that are based, not on a compared list of a half dozen data points, but on a whole computer full of millions of data points, far more information than your conscious mind can process and still maintain sanity.

What if I told you that you had access to a super computer with 5 separate input devices monitoring thousands of bits of information every minute? This computer is constantly comparing all of this input to patterns stored in its memory, evaluating and re-evaluating all the possible options and outcomes. The name of this computer is your brain. The constant stream of live input comes from your five senses; sight, sound, smell, touch and taste. While your front brain is busy driving the car and deciding on where to have lunch, your back brain is busy recording and processing everything in your surroundings.

You're driving along, thinking about what you'd like to have for lunch and suddenly you get a funny feeling in your stomach associated with the car in front of you, a "watch out". While you were thinking about a Ruben sandwich, your brain was noticing that the car in front of you crossed the yellow line twice, the car's speed is erratic, and the driver's head is bobbing. Now that you've been warned you start to consciously notice them and phone 911. That is intuition at work.

How did we develop this reliance on decisions from barely perceived sensory information? Evolutionary biology can offer some interesting clues. I once asked a neurobiologist why the sense of smell is the only one of the five senses with a direct connection to the brain. The answer was in the form of a "what if". What if you were a Neanderthal living in a cave and something was sneaking up on you in the middle of the night with intentions of having you for it's dinner. You're asleep, so sight, touch and taste are on temporary hold. Hearing could help but you would have to assume that creatures that sneak up in the night have gotten good at being silent. What's left would be smell, and, in fact, most things that would like to have you for dinner smell bad. It's entirely possible that the nasty smell would have aroused the Neanderthal in time for him to make his escape and keep the species alive.

My children and I used to go on regular camping/backpacking trips sometimes as far as 20 miles from any civilization. Once in the middle of the night there was a commotion outside the tent. I was pulling on my shoes to go out and see what it was, when my daughter Kim stopped me. She said; "Don't go out there" and after asking her why, she said; "smell it" and there was, in fact, the aroma of rotting meat in the air. I stayed in the tent, the commotion stopped, and in the morning we went out to survey the campsite. There were huge bear footprints all over the campsite. From then on, it became known as "Kim's Rule".

When you're in a new doctor's office, your front brain is trying to make a decision about proceeding with surgery and mentally checking off the Doctor's credentials and attributes. At the same time, your back brain is in hyperdrive, recording and processing sights, sounds, movements in the office, personal interactions, smells, colors, subtle eye movements, and words being said by intonation, innuendo, and body language.

The back brain (intuition) can't announce it's findings like the neon sign in the pizza shop, It only has three messages;

1. Run. – (Major adrenalin rush, the bear is right around the corner.)

2. Everything fits and we're still interested. (Warm and Fuzzy feeling)

3. Something is not right here. (I'm going to warn you by making you uncomfortable and give you that "queasy" feeling in your stomach.)

Learn to listen to these signals and they could save you a lot of pain and suffering or maybe even your life.

Sometimes an intuition can come in just seconds. My wife and I recently visited a new restaurant but, literally, in a few seconds, the queasy uneasy feeling came on. I told her I wanted to leave right away and she reluctantly agreed in spite of violating what she considers proper restaurant protocol. As we're leaving, the couple near the door told us; "good decision, we've been here an hour and they haven't taken our order yet".

Malcolm Gladwell, in his book "Blink" makes the case that a decision (intuition) can come at us so fast, that we tend to doubt it's validity. He uses the term "thin slices" for the amount of time required to make a decision and the "thin slices" may be only a few seconds.

The bad news about intuition is for it to work you must have some knowledge of the subject. If you're counting on your intuition to write a great concerto (like Mozart), an epic poem (like TS Elliot), or discover the secret of matter (like Albert Einstein), your brain must have primed with enough information and data from those fields for the processing to occur. Albert Einstein, a great believer that all great discoveries derive from intuition, had a background in Physics and Mathematics. It's highly unlikely, without some knowledge of Physics, you would have awakened with $E=MC^2$ running around in your head.

When you're driving home and you're struck with the thought that this might be your big chance to win the lottery, that's not intuition. There's no information processing. That decision takes place in a part of the brain sensitive to "urges" like sex, love and lotteries and those urges are probably moderated by chemicals.

The good news, intuition about human-human interactions is built in (if we just listen). Ever since we were infants, we learned that correctly interpreting our parent's moods and emotions would result in love and attention. Throughout our lives we constantly refine and use these intuitions although we sometimes call it "body language". The complete inability to read and respond appropriately to human "body language" or socialization, is a hallmark of Autism, the exact antithesis of intuition.

Going back again to evolutionary biology, a caveman out on a hunting expedition who encounters another hunter would have only a second or two (thin slice) to assess the other hunter for hostility. An incorrect intuition removed him from the gene pool.

"All great men are gifted with intuition. They know without reasoning or analysis, what they need to know."

-- *Alexis Carrel*

"When making a decision of minor importance, I have always found it advantageous to consider all the pros and cons. In vital matter, however, such as the choice of a mate or profession, decisions should come from the unconscious, from somewhere within ourselves. In the important decisions of our personal lives we should be governed by the deep inner needs of our nature."

--*Sigmund Freud*

"The only real valuable thing is intuition."

--*Albert Einstein*

"Have the courage to follow your heart and intuition. They somehow already know what you truly want to become. Everything else is secondary."

--*Stephen Jobs*

"Intuition is always right in at least two important ways;
It is always in response to something.
It always has your best interest at heart."

--*Gavin de Becker,*

"One of our greatest gifts is our intuition. It is a sixth sense we all have – we just need to learn to tap into and trust it."

--Donna Karan, Fashion designer

"The human mind works at low efficiency. Twenty percent is the figure usually given. When, momentarily, there is a flash of greater power, it is termed a hunch, an insight, or intuition."

--Isaac Asimov, Foundation and Empire

"Reason offers us many possibilities at once. Intuition infallibly chooses the best. Remember this and you cannot err; you will always make the right choice."

--Arthur Japin, In Luchis'a Eyes

"I knew immediately something was terribly wrong, but you can know that and not allow the thought in your head, at the front of your head. It dances around at the back, where it can't be controlled."

--Sebastian Barry, The Secret Scripture

"Your mind will answer most questions if you learn to relax and wait for the answer."

--William Burroughs

"Only intuition can protect you from the most dangerous individual of all, the articulate incompetent."

--Robert Bernstein

"The intellect has little to do on the road to discovery. There comes a leap in consciousness, call it intuition or what you will, and the solution comes to you and you don't know how or why.

All great discoveries are made in this way."

--Albert Einstein

Munchausen

Baron Munchausen (Heironymus Carl Friedrich von Münchhausen) was a genuine German adventurer and nobleman. He joined the Russian cavalry in the Russo-Turkish Wars (1735-1739) and achieved the rank of a cavalry captain. He retired in 1760 and returned to his estate in Germany. In his retirement, he acquired a reputation as a teller of highly exaggerated adventure stories. A collection of seventeen tall tales appeared in 1781 which included among the Baron's escapades; ridding a cannonball, a battle with the Turkish army, a balloon expedition to the moon, an encounter with Venus, and being swallowed by a huge sea creature. It has been questioned whether the intent of the Baron was satire and the true meaning of the stories lost to history, but it's equally possible that they were just intended for amusement.

In 1951 A British Physician, Richard Asher described three cases of patients whose disorder led them to falsify medical history, travel from hospital to hospital and even injure themselves to obtain the medical treatment they believed they needed. Asher recommended calling the syndrome Munchausen. "Like the famous Baron von Munchausen, the persons affected have always traveled widely; and their stories, like those attributed to him, are both dramatic and untruthful. Accordingly, the syndrome is respectfully dedicated to the Baron and named after him".

"The Adventures of Baron von Munchausen" is a 1988 British adventure fantasy comedy film written and directed by Terry Gilliam (Monty Python), starring John Neville, Sarah Polley, Eric Idle, Jonathan Pryce, Oliver Reed, Uma Thurman and Robin Williams. The film was caught in a change-of-command at Columbia Pictures and was never properly promoted. Although a box office failure, it can still be found on DVD.

The Monty Hall Paradox

http://www.youtube.com/watch?v=9vRUxbzJZ9Y

The "Monty Hall paradox" is both a perplexing mathematical question and an interesting study of human behavior. It's based on the game show, "Lets Make a Deal" with host Monty Hall. The contestants were asked to choose one of three doors on the stage with a chance of winning either a joke prize or a significant prize. After choosing their door, Monty would open one of the other two doors showing that it contained a joke prize or nothing at all. The contestant was then given the opportunity to change their choice of doors or to stay with the original. The vast majority (over 90%) would stay with their first choice. Not only does this confirm the powerful tendency of people to stick with a decision once it's been made, but the second part of the paradox is just as interesting. Those who mustered the courage to change doors doubled their chances of winning.

Universal Pain Scale

Are you in pain?

0	1 - 2	3 - 4	5 - 6	7 - 8	9 - 10
very happy, I do not hurt at all	hurts just a little bit	hurts a little more	hurts even more	hurts a whole lot	hurts as much as you can imagine, you don't have to be crying to feel this bad

Trust Me, I'm a Plastic Surgeon

Web References

ABMS – American Board of Medical Specialties Home page
  http://www.abms.org

ABMS List of specialties
  http://www.abms.org/who_we_help/physicians/specialties.aspx

ABMS – way to check doctor's certification
  https://www.certificationmatters.org/is-your-doctor-board-certified/search-now.aspx

American Board of Plastic Surgery - Is your surgeon certified?
  https://www.abplsurg.org/ModDefault.aspx?section=SurgeonSearch

Questions from ABPS
  https://www.abplsurg.org/ModDefault.aspx?section=Faq

ASPS – American Society of Plastic Surgery Home page
  http://www.plasticsurgery.org

Overview of Cosmetic Procedures
  http://www.plasticsurgery.org/Cosmetic-Procedures.html

ASAPS – American Society for Aesthetic Plastic Surgery Home page
  http://www.surgery.org

ASAPS – Overview of procedures
  http://www.surgery.org/consumers/procedures

Nurse anesthetists (RN)
  http://www.anesthesianurse.info

Anesthesiology (MD)
  http://www.asahq.org

ISAPS – International Society of Aesthetic Plastic Surgery
  http://www.isaps.org

State Medical Societies (by the AMA)
  http://www.ama-assn.org/ama/pub/about-ama/our-people/the-federation-medicine/state-medical-society-websites.page

FDA – United Stated Food and Drug Administration
  http://www.fda.gov

National Library of Medicine "Medline" for searching topics (free)
  http://www.ncbi.nlm.nih.gov/pubmed/

Phi and the divine ratio in facial beauty
  http://www.facialbeauty.org/divineproportion.html

Facial beauty and Phi
  http://www.beautyanalysis.com

To keep in touch, ask questions, follow our blog, and see updates to the information go to;

www.TrustMeImAPlasticSurgeon.com

About Dr. Kress

Dr. Kress is Board Certified Plastic Surgeon with over 30 years of experience. He is the founder of Plastic Surgery One and the Kress Cosmetic Breast Center. He completed both a General Surgery internship and a General Surgery residency at the Milton S Hershey Medical Center. This was followed by a two year Plastic Surgery residency before gaining his board certification from the American Board of Plastic Surgery in 1982. He also completed a Microsurgery Fellowship in San Francisco working with the legendary Ralph K Bunke, MD. Dr. Kress is an active member of The American Society of Plastic Surgery, The American Society of Aesthetic Plastic Surgery, The prestigious International Society of Aesthetic Plastic Surgery, The American Society for Lasers in Medicine and Surgery, along with local and regional societies. He is on the clinical faculty of the Milton S Hershey Medical Center.

Dr. Kress remains active in research and was one of only a handful of the original clinical researchers for the new and innovative Cohesive Gel (gummy bear) breast implants. His work with these implants resulted in several TV appearances including MTV and Fox5. He remains active in research using ultrasound to treat and prevent capsular contracture, one of the most vexing problems of breast augmentation. He holds the position of Clinical Advisor to several companies involved with the breast industry.

Dr. Kress feels that international participation is essential to keeping current on the latest developments in the field of Plastic Surgery. He was in Brazil when one of the most innovative tummy tuck procedures was first presented and in South Africa when a very successful "mini facelift" was first introduced. To that end, he has participated in educational programs in Russia, Brazil, Turkey, South Africa, Europe, and Canada. He was honored as the only American Plastic Surgeon to be invited to the opening of a new clinic in Georgia (near Russia) by two of his friends Dr's Sulamanidze.

Dr. Kress has a solo practice in Frederick, Maryland primarily specializing in cosmetic surgery and Plastic Surgery repair. He has an excellent reputation for his honest and straightforward approach to his patient's cosmetic surgery goals and a caring, sympathetic approach to the ever-increasing numbers of patients injured by Plastic Surgery.

CPSIA information can be obtained at www.ICGtesting.com
Printed in the USA
BVOW08s1927091114

374143BV00004B/8/P